Echocardiography
in clinical practice

This publication has been supported
by an unrestricted educational grant from

SERVIER

Echocardiography
in clinical practice

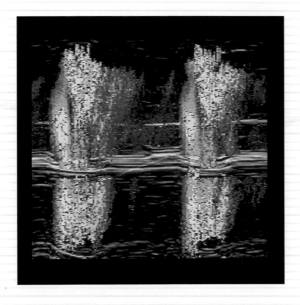

John Chambers MD, FRCP, FESC, FACC

Reader and Consultant in Cardiology
Guy's and St. Thomas' Hospitals, London, UK

The Parthenon Publishing Group
International Publishers in Medicine, Science & Technology

A CRC PRESS COMPANY

BOCA RATON   LONDON   NEW YORK   WASHINGTON, D.C.

**Library of Congress
Cataloging-in-Publication Data**
Chambers, John, MD.
  Echocardiography in clinical practice / John Chambers
      p. ; cm.
  Includes bibliographical references and index
  ISBN 1-84214-108-2 (hardback : alk. paper)
    1. Echocardiography   I. Title
    [DNLM: 1. Echocardiography--methods. 2. Heart diseases--
  diagnosis. WG 141.5.E2 C444e 2001]
  RC683.5.U5 C476 2001
  616.1'207543--dc21

**British Library Cataloguing
in Publication Data**
Chambers, John, 1954–
  Echocardiography in clinical practice
  1.Echocardiography
  I.Title
  616.1'2'07543

ISBN 1842141082

Published in the USA by
The Parthenon Publishing Group
One Blue Hill Plaza, PO Box 1564
Pearl River, New York 10965, USA

Published in the UK and Europe by
The Parthenon Publishing Group
23–25 Blades Court, Deodar Road
London SW15 2NU, UK

Copyright © 2002, The Parthenon Publishing Group
All illustrations © John Chambers

Design and artwork: **randh**design, Lancaster
Printed and bound by T. G. Hostench S.A., Spain

Contents

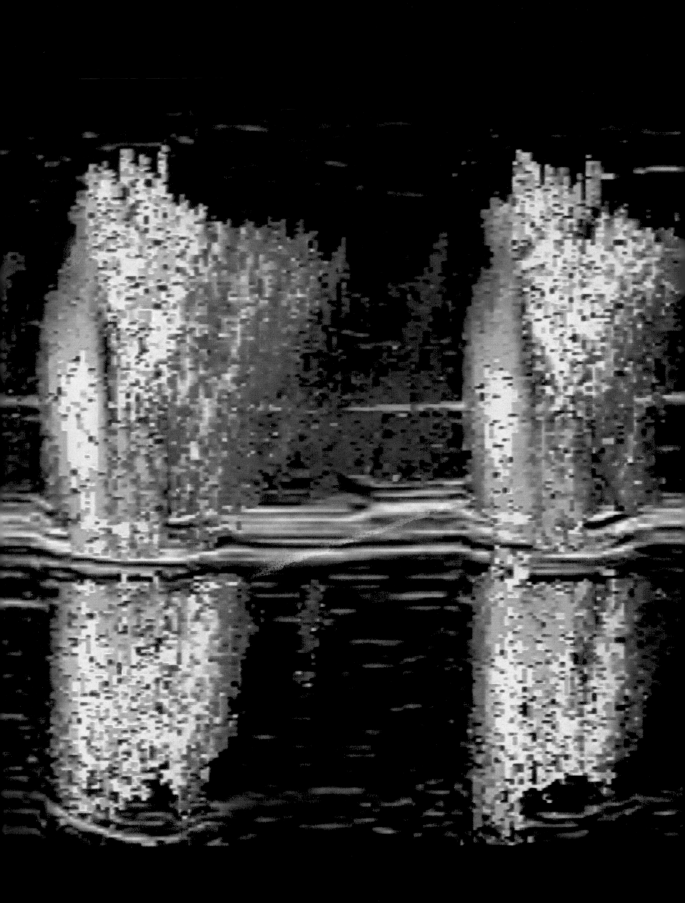

Preface

Most textbooks of echocardiography are systematic treatments from a mainly technical standpoint. The use of echocardiography, however, has long expanded beyond the boundaries of the specialized cardiac unit. General and primary care physicians now request an increasing proportion of studies and need to know what clinical questions modern echocardiography can answer. This short book presents echocardiography from the general clinical perspective. It will also be of use to cardiac specialists in training, who will benefit from a concise overview of the role of echocardiography in cardiac care.

The book is based on *Echocardiography in Primary Care* expanded with chapters based around the recent American College of Cardiology/ American Heart Association guidelines for echocardiography (Cheitlin *et al.*, 1997). Indications for echocardiography were classified as follows:

- Class I: Evidence or general agreement that echocardiography is indicated

- Class IIa: The weight of evidence or opinion favors the use of echocardiography

- Class IIb: Usefulness of echocardiography is less well established

- Class III: Evidence or general agreement that echocardiography is not indicated.

For simplicity, tables have been constructed in which 'indicated' includes classes I and IIa, while 'not indicated' includes classes IIb and III.

Reference

Cheitlin MD, Alpert JS, Armstrong WF, *et al.* ACC/AHA guidelines for the clinical application of echocardiography: executive summary. *J Am Coll Cardiol* 1997;**29**:862–79

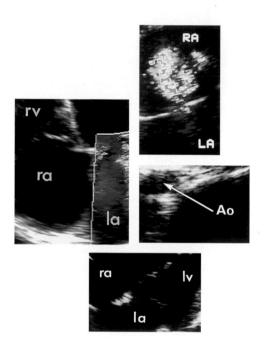

Key to figure abbreviations

Ao	aorta
ASD	atrial septal defect
Cx	circumflex artery
LA, la	left atrium
LAD	left anterior descending artery
LV, lv	left ventricle
P	pericardium
PA	pulmonary artery
PW	posterior wall
RA, ra	right atrium
RCA	right coronary artery
RV, rv	right ventricle
S	septum
VSD	ventricular septal defect

Chapter 1

Echocardiographic techniques

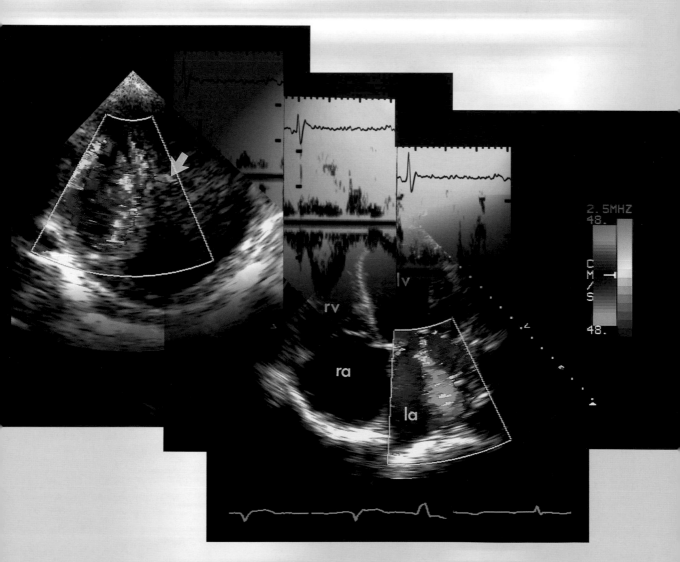

Echocardiography provides information about the anatomy and physiology of the heart. It can detect and quantify the severity of most congenital or acquired heart disorders, and may suggest an etiology. Echocardiography includes both imaging (two-dimensional and M-mode), and Doppler modalities (continuous wave, pulsed, and color flow mapping). These all rely on the piezoelectric effect in which a crystal is made to vibrate by the passage of an electric current. This generates ultrasound waves which are transmitted into the body, with a small proportion being reflected back. The modalities, which can be used separately

Table 1.1 Modalities of echocardiography and their uses

Two-dimensional imaging	Describes anatomy and motion
	Measures left ventricular cavity size and wall thickness if the M-mode cursor cannot be placed perpendicular to the septum and posterior wall
	Measures left ventricular outflow tract diameter for the calculation of stroke volume
	Estimates left ventricular volumes and ejection fraction
	Planimetry of the orifice of the mitral valve in mitral stenosis
M-mode	Measures left ventricular cavity size and wall thickness
	Estimates left ventricular mass
	Times events within the heart
	In combination with color flow mapping aids timing of a flow pattern
Continuous wave Doppler	Calculates the grade of stenotic valve lesions
	Estimates pulmonary artery pressure
	Semiquantitative assessment of the grade of valve regurgitation
Pulsed Doppler	Assesses diastolic left ventricular function from recording at the mitral valve and in a pulmonary vein
	Estimates orifice area of the aortic valve (in combination with two-dimensional imaging and continuous wave Doppler)
	Calculates stroke volume and cardiac output
	Estimates shunt size
Color flow mapping	Screens for abnormal flow e.g. valve regurgitation or a shunt
	Semiquantitative estimate of the grade of valve regurgitation

or together (Table 1.1), differ most in the way that the reflected ultrasound is collected and analyzed.

Two-dimensional echocardiography

Most of a transmitted pulse of ultrasound is scattered or absorbed, but a little is reflected at interfaces between tissues of different density, for example between right ventricular blood and septal endocardium (Figure 1.1, arrow). Reflected ultrasound distorts the piezoelectric crystal and produces an electric current, the size of which controls the density of a spot on the display screen. The position of this spot

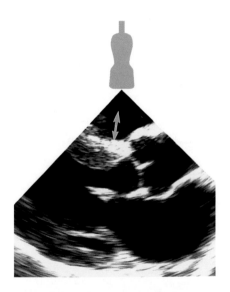

Figure 1.1 Two-dimensional echocardiogram illustrating reflection of ultrasound from the right ventricular cavity/endocardial interface. The transducer position is always at the apex of the image (as illustrated)

is determined by the time difference between transmission and return of the ultrasound. After allowing enough time to collect reflected ultrasound from the deepest parts of the heart, a further pulse is transmitted along the next scan line.

The ultrasound beam moves either by rotation of a mechanical head, or more usually by electronic steering. Substantial processing is carried out within the equipment to compensate for problems such as attenuation of the signal, or divergence of the scan lines.

Current digital machines have increasingly fast processors allowing the handling of immense quantities of data. They do not require conversions between analog and digital formats, so that images on the screen or stored on electronic or optical disk contain all the ultrasound information of the original signal. This means that changes – in depth, sweep-speed or scale, for example – can be made after the original recording. Digital archiving allows rapid comparison with previously recorded images and laboratories are increasingly forgoing paper and tapes.

New technologies, particularly second harmonic imaging, have greatly improved endocardial delineation by two-dimensional echocardiography (Figure 1.2). Second harmonic imaging is now regarded as standard. It relies on the fact that when ultrasound is transmitted through tissue, the waveform is gradually distorted and sends back to the transducer harmonics as well as the original signal. The transducer is set to receive reflected ultrasound at twice the frequency of the transmitted ultrasound. This produces better endocardial definition and fewer artifacts at the price of lower resolution. It is also important to remember that second harmonic imaging makes valves look thicker and may increase septal width, leading to possible overdiagnosis of left ventricular hypertrophy.

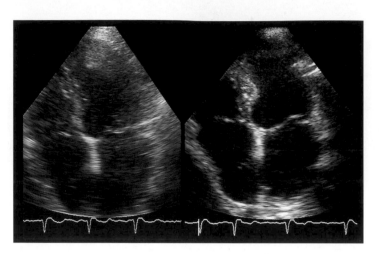

Figure 1.2 Second harmonic imaging. An apical four-chamber view is shown in fundamental (**left**) and second harmonic imaging (**right**). Artifacts (e.g. reverberation and side-lobes) are reduced, allowing better endocardial definition at the expense of lower resolution

Two-dimensional echocardiography is applied for the following purposes:

- To describe anatomy and motion. For example it can show whether an aortic valve has two instead of three cusps and then how well the valve opens. It shows whether the left ventricular shape is normal and how well each part of the wall thickens

- To measure cavity size and wall thickness

- To measure left ventricular outflow tract diameter for the calculation of stroke volume

- To estimate left ventricular volumes and ejection fraction

- Planimetry of the mitral valve orifice in mitral stenosis.

M-mode echocardiography

M-mode stands for motion mode. An M-mode recording (Figure 1.3) is constructed by transmitting and receiving ultrasound along only one scan line, thus giving substantially greater sensitivity than two-dimensional echocardiography for recording moving structures. The returning echoes are displayed as a graph of depth against time.

M-mode can only be applied accurately if the cursor can be aligned perpendicularly to the structure being

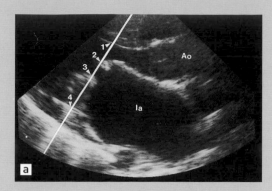

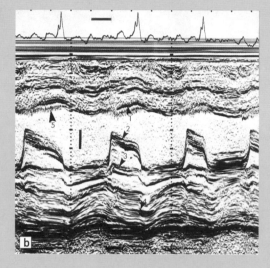

Figure 1.3 M-mode and two-dimensional echocardiograms in a patient with rheumatic mitral stenosis. An M-mode scan line has been chosen through the tips of the mitral leaflets. The following structures may be seen on both the two-dimensional (**a**) and M-mode image (**b**): left septal echo (**1**); tip of anterior mitral leaflet (**2**); posterior leaflet (**3**); and posterior left ventricular wall (**4**). There is also vibration of the left septal echo as a result of coexistent aortic regurgitation (**5**). In the M-mode image, the vertical bar represents 1 cm and the horizontal bar 200 ms

Figure 1.4 The Doppler principle. Red blood cells moving towards the transducer cause a contracted wavelength (velocity displayed above the line); red blood cells moving away from the transducer cause a drawn-out wavelength (velocity displayed below the line)

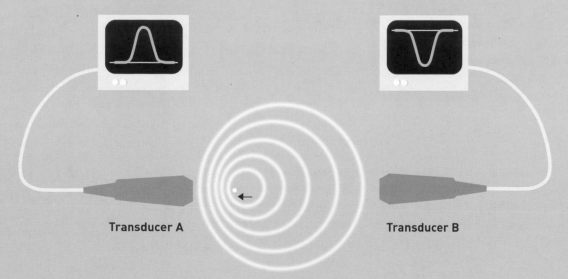

Transducer A　　　　　　　　　**Transducer B**

Figure 1.5 Continuous wave recording in pulmonary stenosis, showing velocity (m/s) and time (msec) on the vertical and horizontal axes, respectively. The signal has been recorded from the left parasternal position. The dense part of the signal (**arrow**) is mainly from blood moving within the right ventricle; the high-velocity signal is from blood passing through the stenotic valve

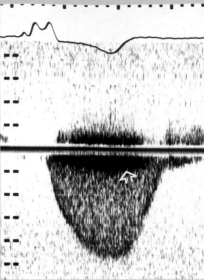

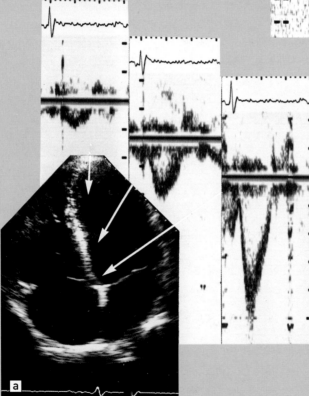

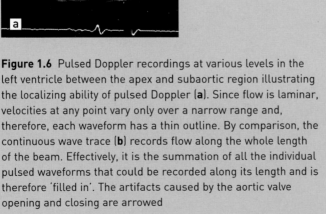

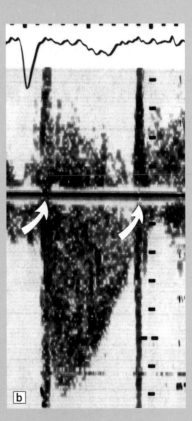

Figure 1.6 Pulsed Doppler recordings at various levels in the left ventricle between the apex and subaortic region illustrating the localizing ability of pulsed Doppler (**a**). Since flow is laminar, velocities at any point vary only over a narrow range and, therefore, each waveform has a thin outline. By comparison, the continuous wave trace (**b**) records flow along the whole length of the beam. Effectively, it is the summation of all the individual pulsed waveforms that could be recorded along its length and is therefore 'filled in'. The artifacts caused by the aortic valve opening and closing are arrowed

assessed. This is now possible in any angulation on a frozen digitized frame. M-mode is used for:

- Measurement of cavity size and wall thickness

- Estimation of left ventricular mass

- Timing of events within the heart e.g. Q wave to mitral valve opening as a measure of diastolic function

- Aiding timing of a flow pattern in combination with color Doppler.

Continuous wave Doppler

In the main Doppler modalities, ultrasound is reflected from moving red blood cells. The Doppler principle is then used to derive velocity information from the frequency shift that occurs between transmitted and reflected ultrasound. The frequency shift (Δf) is twice the transmitting frequency ($2.f_O$) multiplied by the blood velocity corrected for angle ($v.\cos\theta$) and divided by the speed of sound (c). If red blood cells are moving towards the transducer when they reflect ultrasound, the reflected wavelength will be contracted; if they are moving away, the wavelength will be drawn out (Figure 1.4). Computerized analysis of the returning Doppler signal allows velocity and direction to be encoded. By convention, velocities towards the transducer are displayed above the line, and away from it below the line.

A continuous wave Doppler transducer consists of two crystals, one transmitting continuously, the other receiving continuously. The Doppler frequency shift is in the audible range, and the audio signal is used to guide the transducer to obtain the best visual display. This display is a graph of velocity against time, with an additional densitometric dimension because the density of any spot is related to the number of red cells moving at that velocity. For example, in a recording from the left intercostal space with the transducer aimed towards a stenotic pulmonary valve, the display is most dense near the baseline (Figure 1.5, arrow), reflecting the fact that most of the blood above and below the valve is moving at a low velocity (about 1 m/s). Blood accelerating through the valve is at higher velocities, up to 5 m/s.

Continuous wave Doppler is used to estimate the severity of valve stenoses and pulmonary artery pressure and can give a semiquantitative assessment of regurgitation (see also Figures 4.13 and 4.15). The technique can measure high velocities, but is limited by being unable to localize a flow signal, which could originate from anywhere along the length and width of the ultrasound beam.

Pulsed Doppler

The need to localize a flow disturbance, or to record velocity information from a relatively small region, led to the development of pulsed Doppler. A single crystal transmits and then receives ultrasound after a preset time delay. Reflected signals are recorded only from a depth corresponding to half the product of the time delay and the speed of sound. This modality is usually combined with two-dimensional imaging in the same transducer, so that the region where velocities are measured can be localized approximately by placing a 'sample volume' over the image on the screen

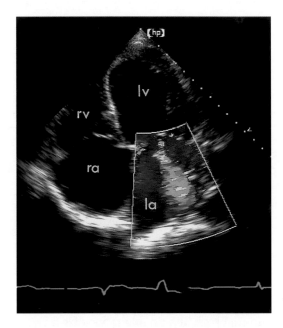

Figure 1.7 Color flow map showing mitral regurgitation. This is an apical four-chamber view in a patient with an anterior infarct. There is a jet of mitral regurgitation within the left atrium

(Figure 1.6). Pulsed Doppler is mainly used to describe diastolic behavior of the left ventricle (see also Figures 2.8 and 3.7), and to calculate stroke volume for use in the calculation of effective valve orifice area (see also Figure 4.11), cardiac output (see also Figure 3.5) and intracardiac shunts. Because the time delay limits the rate at which a waveform can be sampled, there is a limit to the maximum velocity that can be detected accurately.

Color flow Doppler mapping

Color flow mapping is effectively an automated two-dimensional version of pulsed Doppler and calculates mean blood velocity and direction of flow at multiple points down a scan line. Using color encoding, the velocity information is then superimposed on the image (Figure 1.7). By convention, velocities towards the transducer are displayed in red, and those away in blue. Increasing velocities are shown initially in progressively lighter shades, or changes of hue. Above a threshold velocity, a reversal of color occurs, which aids visual detection of abnormal flow. Thus, a mitral regurgitation jet in the left atrium appears blue with some additional yellows. Sometimes a pixel where there is a wide range of velocities is depicted in green which highlights turbulence or regions of high flow acceleration.

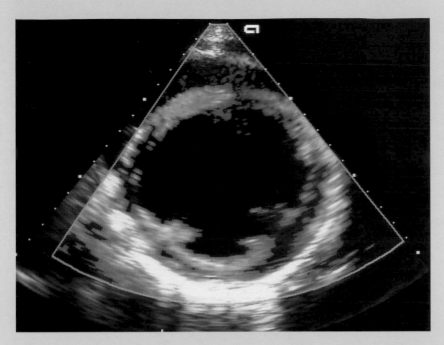

Figure 1.8 Doppler tissue imaging. This is a map of Doppler velocities derived from myocardium. Various components can be encoded, including velocity (as in this example), acceleration or intensity of the signal. This display allows screening for abnormalities of wall motion amplitude or phase to be detected

Figure 1.9 Doppler tissue imaging. Pulsed Doppler allows localization and quantification of motion. In this normal subject, the pulsed sample has been placed on the septal side of the mitral annulus. There is motion towards the apex in systole (**arrow**) and away in diastole

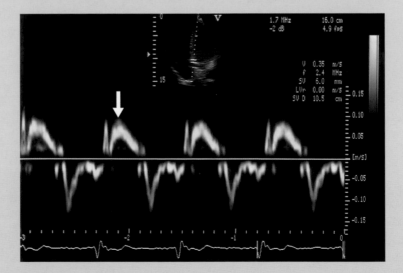

Color mapping is used as a screening tool for abnormal blood flow, particularly regurgitant jets or shunts. It can also give a semiquantitative estimate of the severity of regurgitation (see also Figures 4.11 and 4.15).

Doppler tissue imaging

Color flow mapping assigns colors to different velocities within the blood pool. Doppler tissue imaging does the same for the myocardium, from which the signals have lower velocity but higher amplitude than from the blood pool. Therefore for Doppler tissue imaging, the high-pass filter which normally screens out high-amplitude signals arising from the wall is bypassed and the gain is lowered to eliminate the low-amplitude signals from the blood pool. This gives a display which is superficially like a colorized two-dimensional or M-mode image (Figure 1.8), but in which the information is Doppler-derived. It is possible to detect gradients of velocity within the myocardium. Using a pulsed sample, the velocity pattern at any point in the myocardium or at the mitral (Figure 1.9) or tricuspid annulus throughout the cycle can be displayed. This is being explored for describing regional systolic and diastolic function. Doppler tissue imaging is still largely an experimental technology but is likely to be useful for:

- Detecting asynchrony of contraction e.g. early depolarization in Wolff–Parkinson–White syndrome or the origin of ventricular tachycardia

- Describing diastolic and systolic function including time intervals, regional function, long axis function and differences between endocardial and epicardial function. These can be used for the diagnosis of coronary disease at rest or during dobutamine stress.

Transesophageal echocardiography

In echocardiography there is always a trade-off between attenuation and resolution. Lower frequency transducers, as required for most transthoracic imaging, have good penetration, but relatively poor resolution. The trans-esophageal approach has the advantage that the esophagus is close to the base of the heart which means that attenuation of ultrasound is small and a relatively high frequency transducer can be used, mounted on a modified gastroscope. Furthermore, structures like the descending thoracic aorta or atria, which are distant from the chest wall and therefore hard to image transthoracically, are closely adjacent to the esophagus. A mechanical valve in the mitral position shields the left atrium

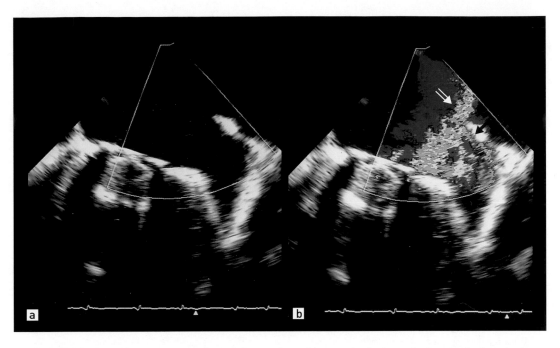

Figure 1.10 Transesophageal echocardiogram in a patient with a mechanical prosthetic valve in the mitral position. There is a large paraprosthetic jet dividing into two with one branch remaining in the left atrium (⇒) and the other entering the left atrial appendage (→)

which prevents ultrasound entering from the transthoracic approach, but this is not a problem via the 'back door' approach (Figure 1.10). The disadvantage of transesophageal echocardiography is that it is obviously more invasive, time-consuming and uncomfortable for the patient than transthoracic echocardiography. It is often seen as better than transthoracic echocardiography because the image quality is usually better. However, the two techniques are complementary. Transthoracic echocardiography is better for imaging the apex of the left ventricle and also the anterior aortic wall

and inferior vena cava, and often the upper part of the ascending thoracic aorta. By contrast the transesophageal approach is better for the atria, pulmonary veins and descending thoracic aorta. Transesophageal echocardiography is now used routinely during cardiac surgery to monitor left ventricular wall motion, de-airing of the heart and the results of valve repair. It is also used for high-risk patients having non-cardiac surgery to assess left ventricular function and to detect the development of myocardial ischemia. On intensive care units transesophageal echocardiography

Table 1.2 Indications for transesophageal echocardiography
(with preparatory transthoracic study)

Suspected endocarditis
- In all cases of prosthetic valve endocarditis
- If the transthoracic study is nondiagnostic
- Consider in all cases of native aortic endocarditis

Cerebral infarction, transient ischemic attack, peripheral embolism
- Patients aged < 50 years with cerebral infarction
- Patients aged > 50 years without evidence of cerebrovascular disease or other obvious cause, in whom the findings of echocardiography will change management (e.g. to start warfarin if a patent foramen ovale is found)

Before cardioversion (under discussion)
- High risk of a cardioembolic event e.g. previous cardioembolic event, or the presence of structural heart disease even if atrial fibrillation is of recent onset
- Anticoagulation contraindicated
- Patients benefitting from early cardioversion e.g. heart failure, inpatients

Prosthetic valve
- If the patient is unwell, even if the transthoracic study is normal
- To improve quantification of mitral regurgitation
- Suspected endocarditis

Native valve disease
- To determine feasibility and safety of balloon mitral valvotomy
- To determine whether some cases of mitral regurgitation are repairable

Atrial septal defect
- To determine whether percutaneous closure is possible

Aorta
- To diagnose dissection, intramural hematoma or transection
- To determine the size of the aorta if not clear transthoracically

Intraoperative
- To monitor left ventricular function
- To assess de-airing of the heart after cardiac surgery
- To assess the result of valve repair

Intensive care unit
- To assess loading, left and right ventricular function and valve function

Poor transthoracic window
- This is a rare indication

is used to assess loading conditions, ventricular function, the presence of pericardial fluid and valve defects.

Stress echocardiography

Stress echocardiography is used to predict the presence of coronary disease, to stratify the risk of a coronary event and to detect hibernation. It is also used for the assessment of functional reserve in patients with end-stage valve disease.

For the detection of coronary disease and stratification of risk, stress echocardiography is similar in accuracy to myocardial perfusion imaging. The sensitivity is slightly lower for echocardiography, but the specificity is slightly higher. The most frequently used stressors are exercise or dobutamine, although some centers use adenosine. Stress echocardiography relies on the fact that abnormalities of relaxation or contraction occur earlier than either chest pain or ST segment changes, so it is more sensitive than conventional electrocardiographic exercise testing. Furthermore, echocardiography can localize the site and quantify the extent of ischemia.

Hibernation occurs either when coronary blood flow falls chronically or as a result of repeated episodes of acute ischemia, so that the myocardium does not have enough energy to contract but is still able to repair wear and tear. This occurs in an uncertain number of patients after myocardial infarction and offers the chance of reversal of left ventricular dysfunction by revascularization. If hibernation is present and the heart is not revascularized, the mortality is far higher than if there is no viability at all. Dobutamine stress echocardiography is similar in sensitivity to positron emission tomography (PET) scanning for the detection of viability. Comparisons with gadolinium-enhanced magnetic resonance imaging are still in progress. The indications for stress echocardiography are given in Table 1.3.

Table 1.3 Indications for stress echocardiography

- Clinical uncertainty and normal or equivocal conventional exercise test
- Patient unable to exercise
- Resting electrocardiogram precluding electrical analysis (e.g. left bundle branch block, left ventricular hypertrophy with strain, digoxin)
- Risk stratification after acute myocardial infarction
- Need to localize site of ischemia
- To assess functional significance of a coronary stenosis in planning angioplasty or surgery
- To detect hibernating myocardium
- To grade aortic stenosis in the presence of a low left ventricle ejection fraction
- To determine if mitral regurgitation develops or worsens during stress

Portable echocardiography

A number of companies have recently introduced miniaturized echocardiography systems capable of being carried on a ward round, when visiting a patient in the intensive care unit or attending an outreach clinic in the community (Figure 1.11). All include two-dimensional imaging and color flow mapping and some have spectral Doppler (continuous wave and pulsed). Most have a memory which can be downloaded to a parent archiving system.

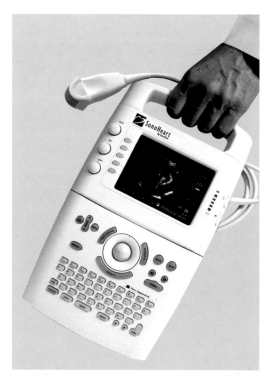

Figure 1.11 Portable echocardiography unit

These systems will extend the clinical examination and promise to open out echocardiography to more patients than can currently be studied by traditional laboratories. The most fruitful applications will probably be the detection of abnormalities of left ventricular or valve function. High-risk groups, such as patients in the community who report breathlessness, can be screened and those found to be abnormal referred to the traditional laboratory for more detailed study. Important issues surrounding training and accreditation need to be addressed since their cost puts these systems within the reach of non-specialist and relatively inexperienced operators.

Further reading

Weyman AE. *Principles and Practice of Echocardiography*, 2nd edn. Washington, DC: Lea and Febiger, 1993

Erbel R, Nesser HJ, Drozdz J. *Atlas of Tissue Doppler Echocardiography TDE*. New York: Springer, 1995

Marwick TH. *Stress Echocardiography*. Dordrect: Kluwer, 1994

Becker H, Burns P. *Handbook of Contrast Echocardiography*. New York: Springer, 2000

Oh JK, Seward JB, Tajik AJ. *The Echo Manual*, 2nd edn. Philadelphia: Lippincott-Raven, 1999

Kerut EK, McIlwain EF, Plotnick GD. *Handbook of Echo-Doppler Interpretation*. New York: Futura, 1996

Chapter 2

The normal heart

Normal ranges and normal variants

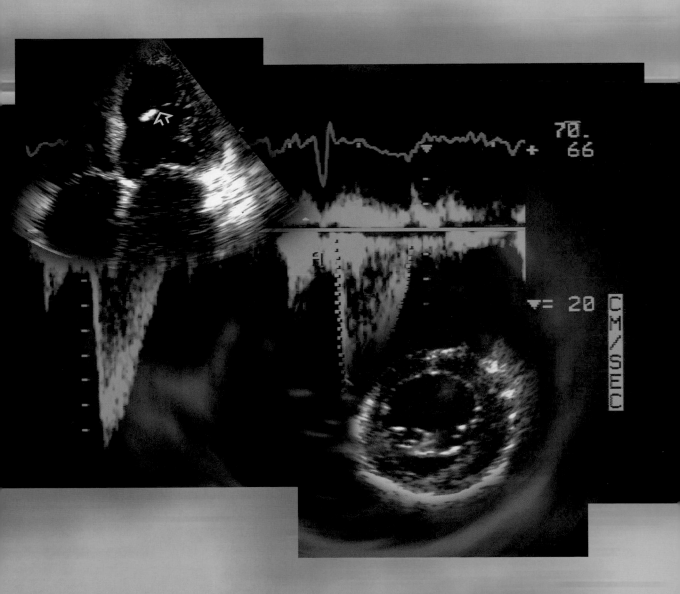

The ribs and lungs mask the heart from ultrasound except at small 'windows' (Figure 2.1) which may be enlarged by asking the subject to lie semirecumbent on his or her left side. The parasternal and apical windows are used routinely.

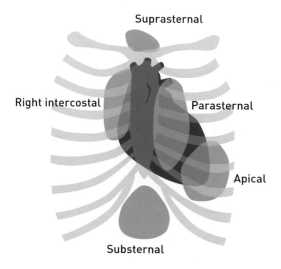

Figure 2.1 The position of the heart and the main echocardiographic 'windows'

The substernal approach is used in patients with lung disease and for imaging the right heart, inferior vena cava, interatrial septum and abdominal aorta; the suprasternal approach is employed mainly for imaging the aorta. The right intercostal approach is used for recording flow across the aortic valve and occasionally for specialized views, particularly of the ascending aorta.

Most examinations start with the parasternal long-axis view (Figure 2.2) in which the heart is 'sliced' lengthways from its base and towards the apex. The transducer is then rotated 90° clockwise and, by tilting on an axis between the left hip and the tip of the right shoulder, transverse (or short-axis) sections through the heart can be obtained at any level from the aorta to the apex. Three standard sections are recorded, through the aortic valve (Figure 2.3), at the level of the mitral valve (Figure 2.4), and through the papillary muscles of the left ventricle (Figure 2.5). The apical approach also allows numerous sections including a four-chamber (Figure 2.6), but also two-chamber and long-axis views. Chamber areas or derived volume are most frequently measured using the apical approach.

M-mode recordings are made at the level of the aortic cusps, at the mitral valve and through the left ventricle just below the tips of the mitral valve. Left ventricular cavity size is measured in systole and diastole (Figure 2.7). The fractional shortening is the difference between left ventricular diastolic (LVDD) and systolic dimensions (LVSD) expressed as a percentage of the diastolic dimension: $100 \times (LVDD - LVSD) / LVDD$. This is a measure of the systolic function of the base of the left ventricle but it can be used as a surrogate for the whole left ventricle provided that this has uniform shape and motion (e.g. there is no myocardial infarction or left bundle branch block).

Figure 2.2 Normal parasternal long-axis view in systole and diastole.

1 papillary muscle
2 chordae tendinae
3 anterior mitral leaflet
4 posterior mitral leaflet
5 mitral–aortic fibrosa
6 posterior mitral annulus
7 non-coronary aortic cusp
8 right coronary cusp
9 sinus of Valsalva

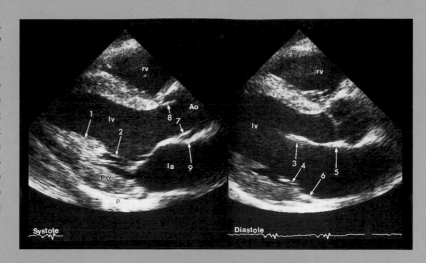

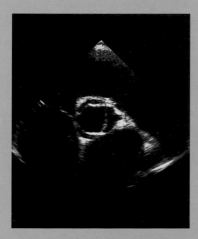

Figure 2.3 Short-axis view at aortic valve level

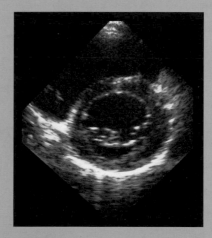

Figure 2.4 Short-axis view at mitral valve level

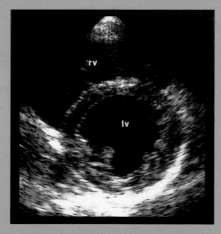

Figure 2.5 Short-axis view at papillary muscle level

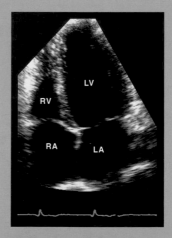

Figure 2.6 Apical four-chamber view

Figure 2.7 Measurement of cavity size on M-mode imaging. Diastolic dimensions and the aorta are measured on the Q wave. The largest left atrial and the smallest systolic left ventricular (**LV**) cavity dimensions are taken.

S septal width
pw posterior wall width
sd systolic LV diameter
dd diastolic LV diameter
Ao aortic diameter
LA left atrial diameter

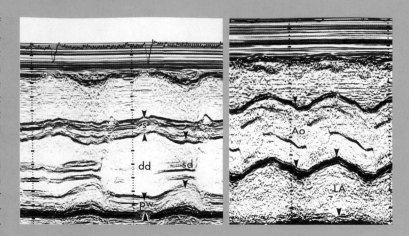

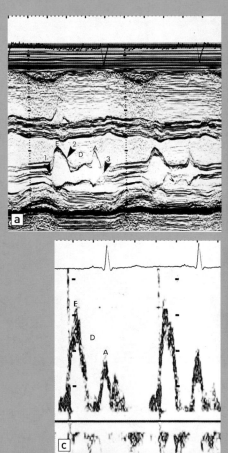

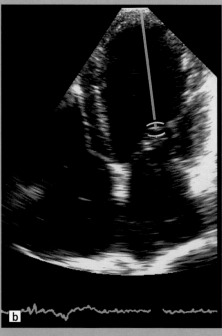

Figure 2.8 (**a**) M-mode recording at mitral valve level; (**b**) position for recording transmitral Doppler; (**c**) transmitral Doppler. The phases of diastole can be seen in (**a**). Initially the mitral valve leaflets open (**1**) at the start of early fast filling (**E**). The leaflets then drift towards the closed position (**2**) during diastasis (**D**) before opening again during atrial systole (**A**). After this the leaflets drift closed (**3**)

Color flow is now turned on as a screen for abnormal flow patterns usually as a result of valve regurgitation, but occasionally from intracardiac shunts. The pulsed Doppler sample is then placed in the left ventricular cavity at the level of the tips of the mitral leaflets in their fully-open diastolic position using the four-chamber view (Figure 2.8). This gives a plot of flow velocities against time. The phases of diastole can be recorded (Figure 2.8): isovolumic relaxation before the mitral valve opens, then early active filling (E). As flow falls after this, the mitral leaflets drift towards the closed position during diastasis (D) and immediately after this the atrium contracts (A).

The sample volume is then turned to record flow through the aortic valve (Figure 2.9). The waveform is effectively a graph of velocity against time and, since distance = speed x time, the area under the curve of the waveform represents the distance travelled in one cycle by blood leaving the left ventricle. This is called the systolic velocity integral or 'stroke distance' and, when multiplied by the cross-sectional area of the left ventricular outflow tract, it gives the stroke volume. The cardiac output is then the product of stroke volume and heart rate.

Normal ranges

Normal dimensions are estimated from small populations of 'average' people and may not apply in unusually small or tall subjects or in the elderly or athletic. This is potentially a major problem if echocardiography is used as a screening tool.

Traditionally, cavity dimensions are measured using M-mode which has better

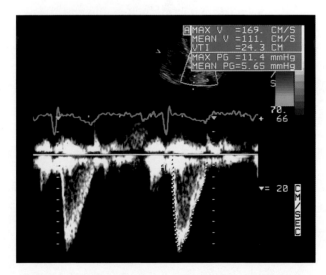

Figure 2.9 Signal recorded in the subaortic area. The pulsed Doppler sample has been placed in the left ventricular outflow tract using the apical approach. The signal has been traced around to measure systolic velocity integral (the same as stroke distance) which is 24.3 cm. Other measures automatically calculated are peak and mean velocity and derived peak and mean pressure difference

resolution than two-dimensional echocardiography. However, despite this theoretical advantage, M-mode imaging may be inaccurate unless the cursor is placed perpendicular to the structure being measured, and this may not always be possible. This is frequently a problem when measuring the aortic root and left atrium when it is common to slice either structure obliquely. Similarly, right ventricular dimensions are inaccurate if measured solely in a parasternal long-axis view. If the cursor cannot be positioned accurately, measurements should instead be made from the two-dimensional images. There is a good case for doing this routinely for the aortic root and left atrium. Gender-specific normal ranges for M-mode measurements are given in Table 2.1. These have been drawn up from the largest available published series and differ from the arbitrary ranges frequently adopted. In particular, the left ventricular dimensions in men are larger than commonly appreciated. Thus,

mild dilated myopathy should not be diagnosed on the basis of an apparently large cavity size alone. Another frequent error is to overestimate the posterior wall width by incorporating chordal echoes in the measurement. Left ventricular hypertrophy should rarely be diagnosed from this measurement alone. Normal ranges for two-dimensional dimensions are given in Figure 2.10. If an accurate assessment of aortic size is required, this should be performed using two-dimensional rather than M-mode echocardiography using the levels shown in Figure 2.11 as a minimum. Normal ranges for aortic size are given in Table 2.2.

Intracardiac dimensions are related to body size and in 'outsize' individuals, it may be difficult to decide if a cavity dimension is normal. It is traditional to index these to body surface area (BSA) although there is good evidence that some dimensions such as the aortic root diameter are better related to height

Table 2.1 Normal intracardiac dimensions (cm) in men and women aged 18–72 years, 150–203 cm (59–80 ins) in height				
	Men		**Women**	
Left atrium	3.0 – 4.5	$n = 288$	2.7 – 4.0	$n = 524$
LV diastolic diameter	4.3 – 5.9	$n = 394$	4.0 – 5.2	$n = 643$
LV systolic diameter	2.6 – 4.0	$n = 288$	2.3 – 3.5	$n = 524$
IV septum (diastole)	0.6 – 1.3	$n = 106$	0.5 – 1.2	$n = 109$
Posterior wall (diastole)	0.6 – 1.2	$n = 106$	0.5 – 1.1	$n = 119$

LV, left ventricular; IV, interventricular and intraventricular. **References:** Lauer MS, Larson MG, Levy D, *et al. J Am Coll Cardiol* 1995;26:1039–46; Devereux RB, Drayer JI, Chien S, *et al. J Am Coll Cardiol* 1984;4:1222–30

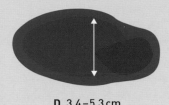
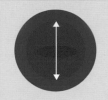
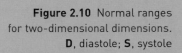

D 3.4–5.3 cm
S 2.3–4.4 cm

D 3.5–6.1 cm
S 2.3–4.1 cm

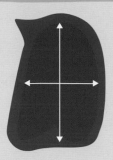

D 3.9–5.9 cm
S 2.7–4.9 cm

D 5.9–9.0 cm
S 4.5–7.9 cm

Figure 2.10 Normal ranges for two-dimensional dimensions. **D**, diastole; **S**, systole

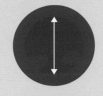

Reference: Pearlman JD, Triulzi MO, King ME, *et al. J Am Coll Cardiol* 1988;**12**:1432–41

D 3.7–6.0 cm
S 2.6–4.4 cm

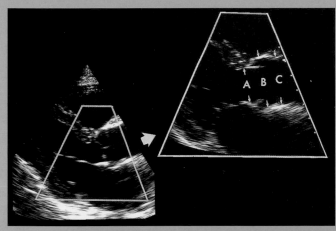

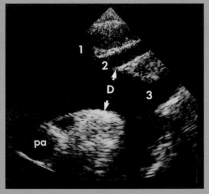

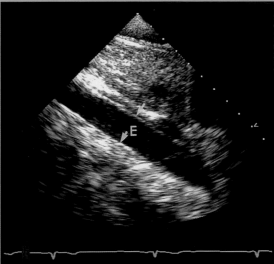

Figure 2.11 The aorta showing levels for measurement.

A annulus
B sinus of Valsalva
C sinotubular junction
D arch
E abdominal aorta
pa pulmonary artery
1 innominate artery
2 left carotid artery
3 left subclavian artery

(Nidorf *et al.*, 1992). M-mode dimensions are given in relation to height in Table 2.3 and two-dimensional dimensions in relation to BSA in Table 2.4.

The elderly are another difficult group since it is not clear whether variations are strictly normal or represent the effect of occult or long-standing mild disease such as hypertension or coronary disease. The elderly tend to have thicker septal and posterior wall widths, but a thickness greater than 1.3 cm is usually abnormal (Klein *et al.*, 1994). Chamber dimensions are variously reported as larger (Pearson *et al.*, 1991) or smaller (Klein *et al.*, 1994) than average, possibly

Table 2.2 Normal ranges (95% confidence intervals) for aortic diameter (cm) using two-dimensional echocardiography

Level (Figure 2.11)	Sample size	Absolute	Indexed to body surface area
A Annulus	*n* = 195	1.7 – 2.5	1.1 – 1.5[1-3]
B Sinus of Valsalva	*n* = 39	2.2 – 3.6	1.4 – 2.0[4]
C Sinotubular junction	*n* = 26	1.8 – 2.6	1.0 – 1.6[5]
D Arch	*n* = 47	1.4 – 2.9	0.8 – 1.9[1]
E Abdominal aorta	*n* = 50	1.0 – 2.2	0.6 – 1.3[1]

References: 1. Unpublished data, Guy's Hospital, London, UK; 2. Oh JK, Taliercio CP, Holmes DR Jr, *et al. J Am Coll Cardiol* 1988;11:1227–34; 3. Davidson WR Jr, Pasquale MJ, Fanelli C. *Am J Cardiol* 1991;67:547–9; 4. Schnittger I, Gordon EP, Fitzgerald PJ, Popp RL. *J Am Coll Cardiol* 1983; 2:934–8; 5. Mintz GS, Kotler MN, Segal BL, Parry WR. *Am J Cardiol* 1979;44:232–8

Table 2.3 Upper limit of intracardiac dimensions (cm) by height (m)

Height	1.41– 1.45	1.46– 1.50	1.51– 1.55	1.56– 1.60	1.61– 1.65	1.66– 1.70	1.71– 1.75	1.76– 1.80	1.81– 1.85	1.86– 1.90	>1.90
M-mode											
Male											
LVDD			5.3	5.4	5.5	5.5	5.6	5.7	5.8	5.9	>6.0
LVSD			3.6	3.7	3.7	3.8	3.8	3.9	3.9	4.0	>4.0
Female											
LVDD	4.9	4.9	5.0	5.1	5.1	5.2	5.3	5.3			
LVSD	3.1	3.2	3.3	3.3	3.4	3.4	3.5	3.5			
Two-dimensional											
Ann	2.0	2.0	2.1	2.1	2.2	2.2	2.3	2.3	2.4	2.4	>2.4
LA	3.2	3.3	3.4	3.4	3.5	3.6	3.6	3.7	3.8	3.9	>3.9

LVDD, left ventricular diastolic dimension; **LVSD**, left ventricular systolic dimension; **Ann**, aortic annulus; **LA**, left atrium
References: Lauer MS, Larson MG, Levy D. *J Am Coll Cardiol* 1995;26:1039–46; Nidorf SM, Picard MH, Triulzi MO, *et al. J Am Coll Cardiol* 1992;19:983–8

Table 2.4 Intracardiac dimensions (cm) on two-dimensional echocardiography by body surface area

		Body surface area (m²)		
		1.4 – 1.6	1.6 – 1.8	1.8 – 2.0
Parasternal long-axis	Diastole	3.4 – 4.9	3.6 – 5.1	3.9 – 5.3
	Systole	2.3 – 3.9	2.4 – 4.1	2.5 – 4.4
Parasternal short-axis mitral level	Diastole	3.7 – 5.4	3.9 – 5.7	4.1 – 6.0
	Systole	2.6 – 4.0	2.8 – 4.3	2.9 – 4.4
Parasternal short-axis papillary	Diastole	3.5 – 5.5	3.8 – 5.8	4.1 – 6.1
	Systole	2.3 – 3.9	2.4 – 4.0	2.6 – 4.1
Four-chamber mediolateral	Diastole	3.9 – 5.4	4.0 – 5.6	4.1 – 5.9
	Systole	2.7 – 4.5	2.9 – 4.7	3.1 – 4.9
Four-chamber long-axis	Diastole	5.9 – 8.3	6.3 – 8.7	6.6 – 9.0
	Systole	4.5 – 6.9	4.6 – 7.4	4.6 – 7.9

Reference: Pearlman JD, Triulzi MO, King ME, *et al. J Am Coll Cardiol* 1988;12:1432–41

Table 2.5 Effect of age on diameter of ascending aorta (cm)

		Height (m)		
Site	Age (years)	1.4 – 1.6	1.6 – 1.8	1.8 – 2.0
Sinus of Valsalva	<40	2.1 – 3.2	2.3 – 3.4	2.5 – 3.6
	>40	2.3 – 3.8	2.3 – 4.0	2.5 – 4.3
Sinotubular junction	<40	1.9 – 2.8	2.0 – 3.0	2.1 – 3.1
	>40	2.1 – 3.3	2.1 – 3.5	2.1 – 3.6

Reference: Roman MJ, Devereux RB, Kramer-Fox R, O'Loughlin J. *Am J Cardiol* 1989;64:507–12

reflecting the presence of different disease states. The aorta is affected differently by age at each level. The annulus is not affected whilst the sinus of Valsalva and sinotubular junction increase in size significantly with age (Table 2.5).

Active athletic individuals may also cause diagnostic confusion. Except in weightlifters, the heart in a trained athlete may be slightly dilated and mildly hypertrophied. The septal width is rarely >1.3 cm and probably never >1.6 cm, but the diastolic cavity dimension may

Table 2.6 Cardiac dimensions (cm) in athletic individuals (95% confidence intervals)

	Male (*n* = 738)	Female (*n* = 209)
LA	3.1–4.3	2.8–4.0
LVDD	4.6–6.2	4.1–5.6
IVS	0.8–1.3	0.7–1.0
PW	0.8–1.1	0.6–1.1

LA, left atrium; **LVDD**, left ventricular diastolic dimension; **IVS**, interventricular septum; **PW**, posterior wall. **Reference:** Pelliccia A, Maron BJ, Spataro A, *et al. N Engl J Med* 1991;**324:** 295–301

Table 2.7 Great vessel peak velocities of blood flow in 110 normal subjects

Site	95% limits (m/s)
Ascending aorta	0.66–1.42
Descending aorta	0.67–1.35
Abdominal aorta	0.47–1.67
Pulmonary artery	0.48–1.16

Reference: Wilson N, Goldberg SJ, Dickinson DF, Scott O. *Br Heart J* 1985;**53:**451–8

be up to 6.2 cm (Pelliccia *et al.*, 1991; Table 2.6). Because it habitually performs at high workload, the left ventricle may be relatively hypocontractile at rest. It is easy to overdiagnose a mild dilated cardiomyopathy in these people.

Normal ranges for Doppler velocities are given in Table 2.7. Relatively high velocities are found in patients with high cardiac output as a result of fever, anemia, pregnancy or anxiety. Ascending aortic velocities of up to 2.0 m/s may be found. Transmitral filling velocities are described in Chapter 3.

Normal variants and technical problems

Most normal variants are obvious but, in the search for pathology in otherwise normal people, these may cause confusion. A large eustachian valve (Figure 2.12) or left ventricular tendon (Figure 2.13) are normal variants which are occasionally misinterpreted as masses. Reverberation artifact (Figure 2.14) may also be overinterpreted as a mass. Technical errors can occur from foreshortening the apex or measuring septal width through a right ventricular papillary muscle to mimic hypertrophy. Another problem is the faithful reporting of small jets of regurgitation, which, to the uninitiated, may suggest pathology. In fact, ultrasound machines are now so sensitive that trivial tricuspid and pulmonary regurgitation are found in virtually all normal subjects and trivial mitral regurgitation may be found in around one-third. However, minor aortic regurgitation is unusual and more likely to be abnormal.

Age-related changes should not be overinterpreted. Minor aortic valve thickening is very frequent and not in

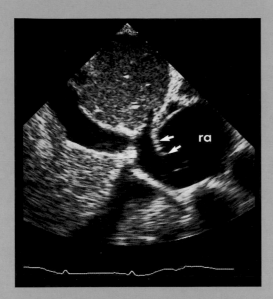

Figure 2.12 Normal variant: large eustachian valve (**arrows**). This valve guards the opening of the inferior vena cava into the right atrium

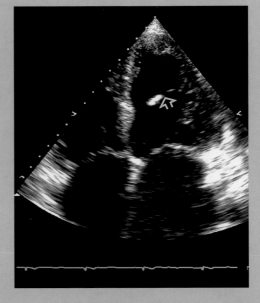

Figure 2.13 Normal variant: left ventricular tendon (**arrow**)

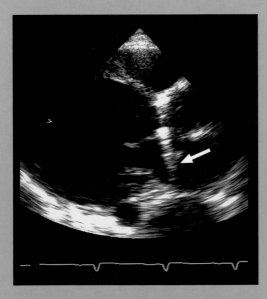

Figure 2.14 Artifact: reverberation artifact from a mechanical prosthetic valve in the aortic position causes the appearance of echoes within the left atrium (**arrow**) which may be mistaken for a mass

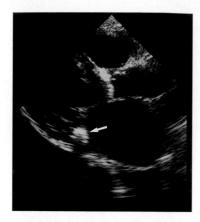

Figure 2.15 Posterior mitral annular calcification (**arrow**)

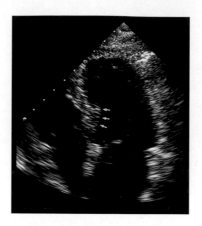

Figure 2.16 Normal variant: localized subaortic bulge (**arrows**)

itself a sign of significant pathology. Mitral annular calcification (Figure 2.15) is occasionally misinterpreted as a vegetation, thrombus or myxoma. Localized subaortic bulging of the septum (Figure 2.16) is normal in the elderly and should not be diagnosed as hypertrophic cardiomyopathy.

References

Klein AL, Burstow DJ, Tajik AJ, *et al.* Effects of age on left ventricular dimensions and filling dynamics in 117 normal persons. *Mayo Clin Proc* 1994;**69**:212–24

Nidorf SM, Picard MH, Triulzi MO, *et al.* New perspectives in the assessment of cardiac chamber dimensions during development and adulthood. *J Am Coll Cardiol* 1992;**19**:983–8

Pearson AC, Gudipati C, Nagelhout D, *et al.* Echocardiographic evaluation of cardiac structure and function in elderly subjects with isolated hypertension. *J Am Coll Cardiol* 1991;**17**:422–30

Pelliccia A, Maron BJ, Spataro A, *et al.* The upper limit of physiologic cardiac hypertrophy in highly trained elite athletes. *N Engl J Med* 1991;**324**:295–301

Schiller NB, Shah PM, Crawford M, *et al.* Recommendations for quantitation of the left ventricle by two-dimensional echocardiography. *Am Soc Echocardiogr* 1989;**2**:358–67

Chapter 3

Suspected heart failure

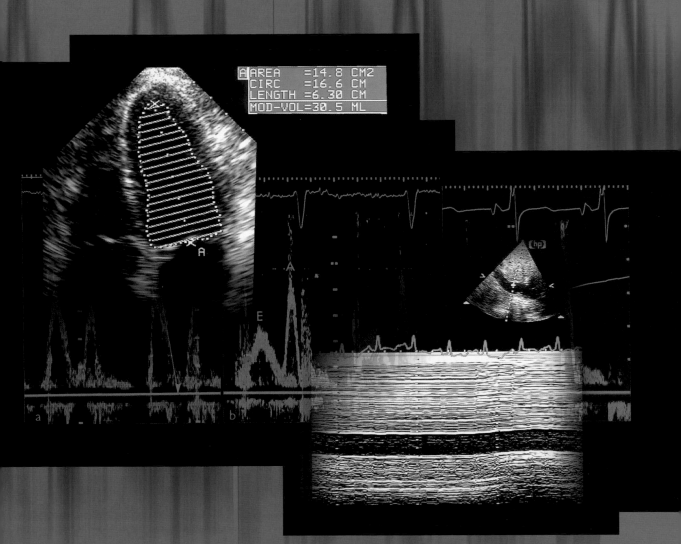

AREA   =14.8 CM2
CIRC   =16.6 CM
LENGTH =6.30 CM
MOD-VOL=30.5 ML

Table 3.1 Indications for echocardiography in suspected heart failure

Indicated

- Breathlessness or dependent edema and clinical findings that suggest or cannot exclude heart disease
- Unexplained hypotension
- Exposure to cardiotoxic agents
- Known cardiomyopathy where there is a change in clinical status

Not indicated

- Routine evaluation in clinically stable patient in whom no change in management is contemplated
- Patients with dependent edema but no evidence of heart disease

effusion or left atrial myxoma, or require specific therapy other than diuretics and ACE inhibitors. For example, valve disease or left ventricular aneurysm may be amenable to surgery.

Heart failure is common, with a prevalence of around 0.4–2% (Cowie *et al.*, 1997). It is not in itself a complete diagnosis. The etiology and underlying pathophysiologic mechanisms need to be determined, as these may affect treatment. For example, as many as 3% of people aged over 75 years may have severe aortic stenosis (Lindroos *et al.*, 1993). If this causes heart failure, the murmur may become inaudible. A proportion of patients with clinical heart failure have predominantly diastolic rather than systolic left ventricular dysfunction (Aurigemma *et al.*, 2001). In these instances, angiotensin converting enzyme (ACE) inhibitors may be either unhelpful or dangerous.

Echocardiography is integral for establishing the diagnosis and pathophysiology (Table 3.1). It is also used to exclude conditions that mimic heart failure such as pericardial

Establishing the diagnosis and pathophysiology

Systolic function

Both regional and global systolic function are examined. Every region corresponding to the arterial supply of the heart (Figure 3.1) is described according to the degree of systolic thickening and by the motion of the endocardium:

- normal
- hypokinetic (the endocardium moves inwards less than 50% of normal) (Figure 3.2)
- akinetic (no motion)
- dyskinetic (motion out of phase with the expected direction) (Figure 3.3).

Global measures of function include ejection fraction, stroke volume, and end-systolic volume. Ejection fraction is usually estimated by eye, but can also be calculated using online computer software. This involves tracing round systolic and diastolic frames, usually in the apical four-chamber and two-chamber views. Systolic and diastolic volumes are calculated using geometric assumptions (Figures 3.4 and 5.4). Stroke volume is then the difference between diastolic and systolic volume and ejection fraction is stroke volume expressed as a percentage of the diastolic volume. However, these calculations are laborious and potentially inaccurate. End-systolic

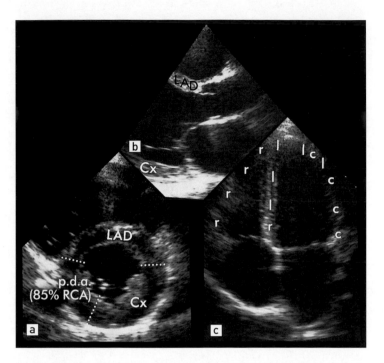

Figure 3.1 The arterial supply of the heart shown in parasternal short axis (**a**), long axis (**b**), and four-chamber (**c**) views. **p.d.a.**, posterior descending artery; **r**, right coronary artery; **l**, left anterior descending; **c**, circumflex

chamber area or derived-volume alone are relatively more accurate because, for technical reasons, the endocardium is

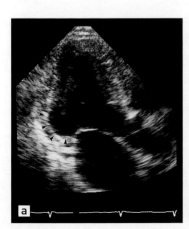 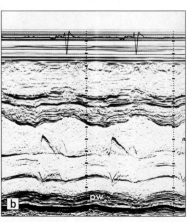

Figure 3.2 Hypokinesis. There is an inferior infarct shown as a bulging region (**arrowed** in **a**). The M-mode recording at this level (**b**) shows hyperkinesis of the septum (**s**) while the inferior wall (**pw**) is hypokinetic

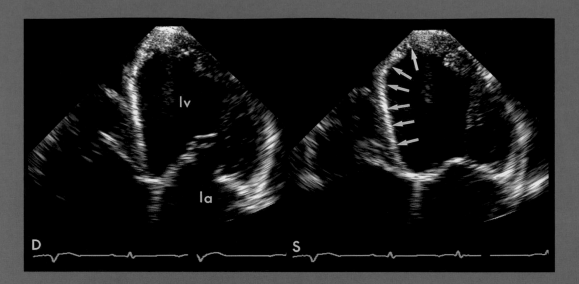

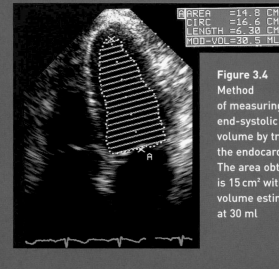

Figure 3.3 Anterior myocardial infarct. The apex and adjacent septum are thin and move paradoxically, i.e. outwards in systole (right, arrows) when the rest of the left ventricle is moving inwards. **D**, diastole; **S**, systole

```
AREA   =14.8 CM2
CIRC   =16.6 CM
LENGTH =6.30 CM
MOD-VOL=30.5 ML
```

Figure 3.4 Method of measuring end-systolic volume by tracing the endocardium. The area obtained is 15 cm² with a volume estimated at 30 ml

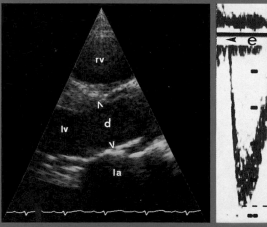

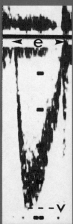

Figure 3.5 Method of estimating stroke volume. This is calculated from the product of the cross-sectional area of the left ventricular outflow tract and the area of the subaortic signal recorded using pulsed Doppler (stroke distance or systolic velocity integral). Note: **d**=diameter; **e**=ejection time; **v**=peak velocity

well imaged in systole. In the diseased heart, there is often a change in shape of the left ventricular cavity even if there is no regional abnormality of movement. Therefore, these end-systolic quantities often reflect the true size of the heart better than do M-mode dimensions. Stroke volume can also be calculated from the product of the cross-sectional area of the aorta and the area of the pulsed Doppler signal recorded in the left ventricular outflow tract (Figure 3.5). This is accurate and compares favorably with thermodilution methods. Normal ranges are given in Table 3.2.

It is important to allow for the effects of loading and drugs when making an assessment of systolic function. Negatively inotropic drugs, such as antiarrhythmic agents, can cause significant reduction in function of an otherwise mechanically normal heart.

Table 3.2 Normal ranges (95% confidence intervals) for measures of systolic and diastolic function

Echocardiography		
Fractional shortening (%)	28–44	
End-diastolic volume (ml)*	58–166 (male)	49–129 (female)
End-systolic volume (ml)*	3–67 (male)	9–57 (female)
Four-chamber area diastole (cm²)	18.6–48.6	
Four-chamber area systole (cm²)	8.6–30.4	
Ejection fraction (%)	50–70	
Doppler		
Systolic velocity integral (cm)	15–35	10–25 (elderly)
Mitral valve E (cm/s)	44–100	34–90 (elderly)
Mitral valve A (cm/s)	20–60	31–87 (elderly)
E:A ratio	0.7–3.1	0.5–1.7 (elderly)
Tricuspid valve E (cm/s)	20–50	
Tricuspid valve A (cm/s)	12–36	
E:A ratio	0.8–2.9	
Time intervals		
Mitral E deceleration time (ms)	139–219	138–282 (elderly)
Mitral A deceleration time (ms)	>70	
Isovolumic relaxation time (ms)	54–98	56–124 (elderly)

*Single plane four-chamber view. **References:** Van Dam I, *et al. Echocardiography* 1988;5:259–67; Zarich SW, Arbuckle BE, Cohen LR, *et al. J Am Coll Cardiol* 1988;12:114–20; Wilson N, Goldberg SJ, Dickinson DF, Scott O. *Br Heart J* 1985;53:451–8; Wahr DW, Wang YS, Schiller NB. *J Am Coll Cardiol* 1983;1:863–8; Schiller NB, Foster E. *Heart* 1996;75(Suppl 2):17–26; Sagie A, Benjamin EJ, Galderisi M, *et al. J Am Soc Echocardiogr* 1993;6:570–6; Van Dam I, Fast J, de Boo T, *et al. Eur Heart J* 1988;9:165–71; Klein AL, Burstow DJ, Tajik AJ, *et al. Mayo Clin Proc* 1994;69:212–24; Rawles J. *Echocardiography: an International Review.* 1993;23–36; Pearlman JD, Triulzi MO, King ME, *et al. J Am Coll Cardiol* 1988;12:1432–41

In the presence of severe mitral regurgitation, the ejection fraction may be normal despite intrinsically reduced contractility. This is because the left ventricle contracts partly into the left atrium which offers much less resistance than the aorta and systemic circulation. It is a little like being treated with large doses of ACE inhibitors. After mitral surgery, the left ventricle is then subject to normal afterload and the ejection fraction falls (Figure 3.6). Conversely, in severe aortic stenosis, the ejection fraction may be low despite normal intrinsic contractility since the left ventricle has to overcome the high transaortic resistance as well as eject blood. After aortic valve replacement measurements of systolic function often improve substantially or revert to normal.

Diastolic dysfunction

Diastolic dysfunction is suggested by the presence of left ventricular hypertrophy in a patient with breathlessness or by abrupt cessation of filling shown as a jerky diastolic motion on two-dimensional imaging. More specific evidence is found from abnormalities of transmitral flow recorded using pulsed Doppler (Figure 3.7) (Cohen *et al.*, 1996). In the normal person, the early velocity (E wave) is higher than the velocity during atrial systole (A wave) and the E descent is quick. There are two main pathologic patterns (Figure 3.7). The first is called the 'slow relaxation pattern' and consists of a low E wave, prolonged E wave deceleration time (and isovolumic relaxation time) with a tall A wave. This pattern is seen in hypertrophied left ventricles. The second pattern is the 'restrictive pattern' which occurs in left ventricular dysfunction from any cause associated with high filling pressures (pulmonary wedge pressure > 20 mmHg) and with a fast rate of rise of left ventricular diastolic pressure (as in restrictive myopathy or pericardial constriction). This has a tall E wave, short E deceleration time (and short isovolumic relaxation time) with a small or absent A wave. Other signs of abnormal diastolic function are a dilated inferior vena cava or abnormal patterns of pulmonary, superior vena cava or hepatic vein flow. For example an abnormally increased peak velocity or duration of atrial flow reversal on pulmonary venous flow recordings suggests elevated end-diastolic left ventricular pressure.

Surgically correctable diseases, mainly pericardial constriction, must first be excluded by advanced echo-cardiographic techniques, sometimes supplemented by computed tomography and cardiac catheterization.

Right-sided disease

Right-sided failure is shown by a dilated, hypokinetic right ventricle. This may be difficult to detect, but, if the right

Figure 3.6 M-mode recordings through the left ventricle before and after mitral valve surgery. The fractional shortening before surgery (**a**) was 29% and afterwards (**b**) was 15%

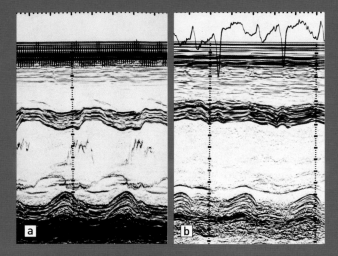

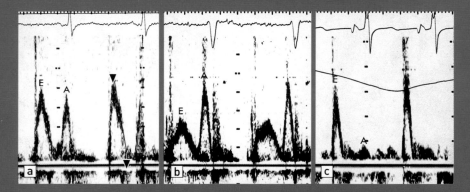

Figure 3.7 Transmitral pulsed Doppler recordings. These were all recorded with the sample volume positioned as shown in Figure 2.8. The patterns are normal (**a**), slow filling (**b**), and restrictive (**c**). The method of measuring the deceleration time of the E wave is shown in **a** (between the two arrows)

Figure 3.8 Dilated inferior vena cava. The diameter should be less than 2 cm and there should be constriction by at least 50% during inspiration. In this image, the diameter remains constant. This is a sign of a raised right atrial pressure, in this case caused by pericardial constriction

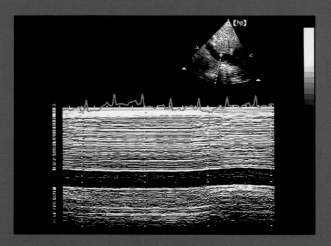

ventricle is the same size or larger than the left ventricle in all views, it must be abnormal. Dilatation of the inferior vena cava (Figure 3.8) indicates high right-sided pressures as a non-specific sign of left or right ventricular failure or pericardial disease. The indications for echocardiography in pulmonary disease are given in Table 3.3.

Table 3.3 Echocardiography in pulmonary disease
Indicated
• Confirmation of suspected pulmonary hypertension and evaluation of response to treatment
• Suspected cor pulmonale
• Breathlessness of uncertain etiology
Not indicated
• Lung disease with no suspicion of cardiac involvement
• Re-evaluation of the right heart with no change in the clinical state

Can we define criteria for diagnosing heart failure?

There are no simple universal criteria and these will depend on the level of suspicion based on the clinical findings. The presence of clinical signs of heart failure and the absence of other causes of breathlessness suggests a high clinical suspicion of heart failure. The presence of breathlessness alone denotes a lower level of suspicion and demands a higher grade of abnormality on the echocardiogram before a working diagnosis of heart failure should be made.

Tables 3.4 and 3.5 give guidelines for determining the likelihood of clinical heart failure. These are to some degree arbitrary, but are based on normal ranges.

Too simplistic a differentiation between diastolic and systolic heart failure is misleading. Systole and diastole are part of a continuous cardiac cycle and interactions between them occur. Mild systolic dysfunction may cause an alteration in the timing of early diastolic events to maintain stroke volume. In a dyskinetic heart, regions can continue contracting into diastole after closure of the aortic valve, leading to a shortening of the time available for left ventricular filling. Conversely, a poorly compliant left ventricle that fails to fill adequately in diastole may cause a low stroke volume in systole.

If clinical doubt remains, the patient must be seen by a cardiologist. **In the**

Table 3.4 Significant left ventricular systolic dysfunction suggesting that heart failure is the likely cause of symptoms
• Ejection fraction <40%
• End-systolic volume >70 ml or 45 ml/m^2
• Fractional shortening <23%
• Stroke distance <10 cm
• Extensive regional wall motion abnormality

Table 3.5 Suggested diagnosis of diastolic heart failure		
	Age <50	**Age >50**
1. E:A ratio and	<1.0	<0.5
E deceleration time	>220 ms	>280 ms
2. S:D ratio	>1.5	>2.5

E:A ratio, early-to-atrial peak velocity ratio on the transmitral signal; S:D systolic/ diastolic peak velocity on the pulmonary vein flow signal. **Reference**: European Study Group on diagnostic heart failure. *Eur Heart J* 1998;**19**:995–1003

presence of a normal echocardiogram, the heart may still be a cause for breathlessness as a result of systolic failure on exertion, diastolic dysfunction or angina. Diastolic dysfunction is difficult to diagnose except by experienced echocardiographers.

Should all patients on antifailure medication be screened?

Preliminary reports suggest that over one-half of all patients taking diuretics or ACE inhibitors have no evidence of a left ventricular systolic abnormality at rest. Allowing for cases with hypertension, treatment with diuretics was judged to be inappropriate in 44% of cases in one study (Francis *et al.*, 1995). However, this underplays the importance of diastolic dysfunction. Furthermore, the echocardiogram may not always reflect the pretreatment state of the patient. Minor abnormalities of systolic or diastolic function may not be obvious at rest or may be obscured by drug treatment. The drug may even have corrected an

underlying abnormality as, for example, when an ACE inhibitor induces regression of left ventricular hypertrophy. Ideally, the whole clinical history should be reviewed checking for previously documented objective signs, evidence of improvement on therapy, other possible causes of breathlessness or other explanations for clinical signs (e.g. varicose veins for ankle swelling). The echocardiogram should be part of this general clinical review, but should not replace it.

Does a normal electrocardiogram exclude the need for echocardiography?

Recent reports have suggested that it is rare to have an abnormal echocardiogram in the presence of a normal electrocardiogram (Task Force for the Diagnosis and Treatment of Chronic Heart Failure, 2001). Despite their suggestion that echocardiography is not necessary if the electrocardiogram is normal, some 10–15% of patients with normal electrocardiograms have important systolic dysfunction on echocardiography. Furthermore, these studies fail to take account of the frequency of diastolic dysfunction. A common cause of this is left ventricular hypertrophy as a result of hypertension and it is well documented that echocardiography is 5–10 times more sensitive than electrocardiography for the detection of left ventricular hypertrophy (see Chapter 5).

An electrocardiogram is a useful first investigation in patients with breathlessness or clinical heart failure. It may show an arrhythmia such as uncontrolled atrial fibrillation as a likely cause of the symptoms. It may also show the signs of a myocardial infarction in which case the clinician is on firm ground in treating with diuretics and ACE inhibitors. A completely normal electrocardiogram should lead to consideration of other causes of symptoms including lung disease, anemia, obesity or angina. However, if diagnostic doubt remains, echcardiography remains necessary.

Etiology of heart failure

The most frequent etiologies of heart failure are ischemic disease, hypertension and valve disease. Ischemic heart disease is characterized by regional wall motion abnormalities (Figure 3.3). There may be complications of infarction such as left ventricular aneurysm (see also Figure 8.3) or, rarely, ventricular septal rupture (see also Figure 8.4) which is present in 1–2% of all acute infarcts. Hypertensive heart disease is suggested by increased left ventricular mass (see Chapter 5) with either a small or dilated cavity depending on the stage of disease, individual susceptibility to pressure

overload and, possibly, the presence of coronary disease. Dilated cardiomyopathy is shown by an unthickened, dilated, globally hypocontractile ventricle (Figure 3.9). However, idiopathic dilated cardiomyopathy cannot be distinguished echocardiographically from specific causes of left ventricular disease such as high alcohol consumption.

Left ventricular dysfunction secondary to valve disease is easily detected by the presence of anatomical abnormalities of the valve on two-dimensional imaging, together with significant aortic stenosis or aortic or

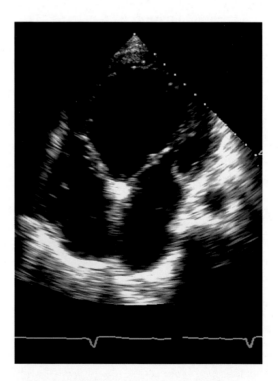

Figure 3.9 Dilated left ventricle in an apical four-chamber view

mitral regurgitation on continuous wave Doppler. The differentiation between severe mitral regurgitation causing left ventricular failure and primary left ventricular myopathy associated with significant functional mitral regurgitation may be difficult.

A combination of two-dimensional imaging and Doppler findings can also detect the causes of right ventricular dysfunction, namely pulmonary hypertension, intracardiac shunts, right-sided valve disease, right ventricular infarction (see also Figure 8.1), and right ventricular cardiomyopathy.

References

Aurigemma GP, Gottdiener JS, Shemanski L, *et al.* Predictive value of systolic and diastolic function for incident congestive heart failure in the elderly: The Cardiovascular Health Study. *J Am Coll Cardiol* 2001;**37**:1042–8

Cohen GI, Pietrolungo JF, Thurmis JD, Klein AL. A practical guide to assessment of ventricular diastolic function using Doppler echocardiography. *J Am Coll Cardiol* 1996;**27**:1753–60

Cowie MR, Struthers AD, Wood DA, *et al.* Value of natriuretic peptides in assessment of patients with possible new heart failure in primary care. *Lancet* 1997;**350**:1349–53

Francis CM, Caruàna L, Kearney P, *et al.* Open access echocardiography in management of heart failure in the community. *Br Med J* 1995;**310**:634–6

Lindroos M, Kupari M, Heikkilä J, Tilvis R. Prevalence of aortic valve abnormalities in the elderly: an echocardiographic study of a random population sample. *J Am Coll Cardiol* 1993;**21**:1220–5

Task Force for the Diagnosis and Treatment of Chronic Heart Failure. Guidelines for the diagnosis and treatment of chronic heart failure. *Europ Heart J* 2001;**22**:1527–60

Chapter 4

The patient with a murmur

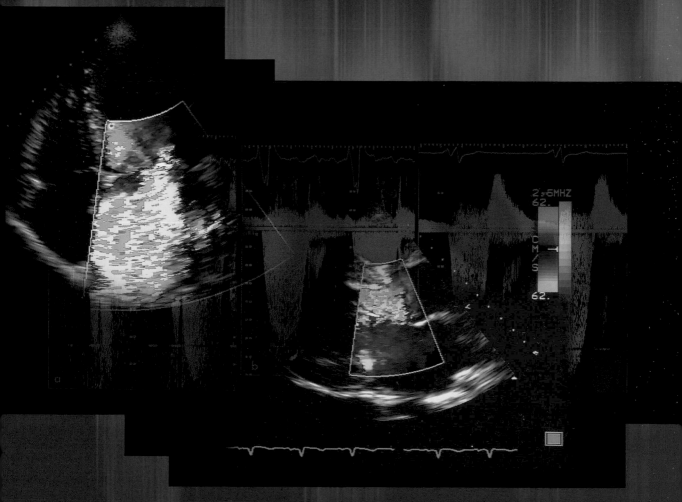

Murmurs are caused by valve disease, an intracardiac shunt or high flow across a normal valve. Echocardiography is necessary if there is the possibility of significant disease (Table 4.1) or to check if antibiotic prophylaxis is necessary. It confirms the site of origin of the murmur by imaging an abnormal valve or detecting abnormal flow on color mapping. It can then reveal the etiology and quantify the severity of disease.

Etiology

The most frequent cause of aortic stenosis in western populations is calcific degenerative disease (Figure 4.1). Minor thickening of the aortic valve is found in 20% of all people aged over 65 years and 40% aged over 75 years (Lindroos *et al.*, 1993). This explains why a short, soft systolic murmur should not automatically require echocardiography. Mild aortic thickening may progress, so the term

Table 4.1 Echocardiography in valve disease

Indicated

- If the patient is previously uninvestigated and symptomatic
- Murmur suggesting at least a moderate probability of organic disease
  - Ejection systolic murmur filling most of systole or any pansystolic murmur
  - Any diastolic murmur
  - Abnormal second heart sound
  - Wide pulse pressure and displaced apex beat or enlarged cardiac shadow
- Re-evaluation if symptoms change or with severe valve disease even with no symptoms
- Re-evaluation if there is left ventricular dilation even if the valve disease is mild or moderate
- Evidence of endocarditis
- Known significant valve disease and pregnancy
- For planning valve replacement, repair or valvotomy
- Routinely soon after valve surgery or if symptoms or signs suggest dysfunction

Not indicated

- Asymptomatic soft ejection systolic murmur and normal second heart sound
- Routine evaluation of asymptomatic patients with mild or definitely moderate aortic or mitral valve disease and normal left ventricular function
- Fever and non-pathologic murmur alone
- Re-evaluation in a prosthetic valve without evidence of dysfunction, endocarditis or left ventricular dysfunction
- Repeat studies in clinically stable endocarditis

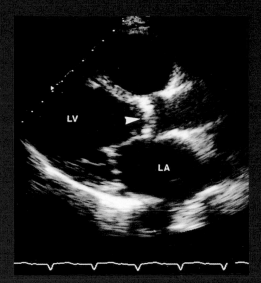

Figure 4.1 Calcific degenerative disease. Parasternal long-axis view (systole). The aortic cusps (**arrow**) should be open but have hardly moved from their closed position in diastole

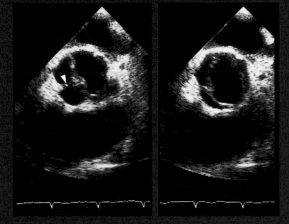

Figure 4.2 Bicuspid aortic valve, diagnosed by the presence of a median raphe (arrow) representing the unseparated cusp edges (transesophageal view: diastole – **left**, systole – **right**)

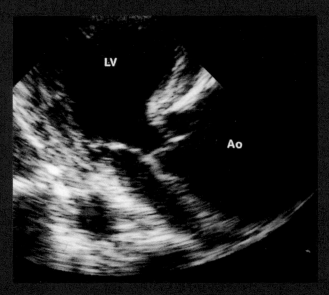

Figure 4.3 Aortic root dilatation (apical long-axis view) in a 75-year-old man with long-standing hypertension

Figure 4.4 Rheumatic mitral stenosis from the parasternal short-axis view. The leaflet tips are thickened and there is a highly echogenic spot (arrow) representing calcification or collagenous thickening where the medial commissure has become fused

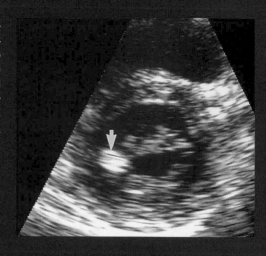

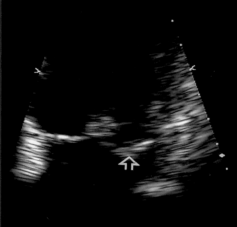

Figure 4.5 Mitral valve prolapse (apical four-chamber view). This view shows curvature of the posterior leaflet (arrow) above the plane of the annulus during systole in the left-hand panel with a broad jet or mitral regurgitation in the right-hand panel

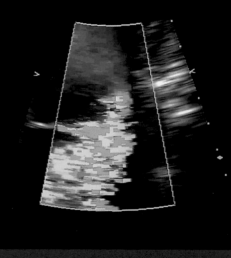

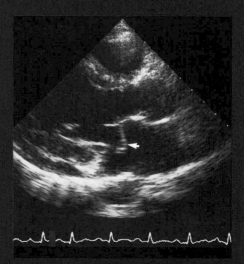

Figure 4.6 Mitral valve vegetation (arrowed) in a 25-year-old woman with fever and malaise

'aortic sclerosis' should be avoided as this is often taken to imply a separate, more benign etiology. A bicuspid aortic valve occurs in around 2% of the population (Figure 4.2), and usually results from failure of two of the cusps to separate during embryologic development. The valve is subject to increased strain and thickens and calcifies more rapidly than usual, leading to significant aortic stenosis typically between 40 and 60 years of age. Aortic regurgitation can be caused either by dilatation of the aortic root or by aortic valve disease, or both. In Western populations, aortic root dilatation (Figure 4.3) is the more frequent cause of significant regurgitation. It usually develops as a result of arteriosclerosis secondary to aging. Of the valve-related causes, rheumatic disease tends to cause more regurgitation than does calcific degeneration as a result of leaflet retraction. Regurgitation may also follow aortic valve destruction in infective endocarditis.

Mitral stenosis is almost exclusively rheumatic in origin (Figure 4.4). Mitral regurgitation is usually caused by left ventricular impairment leading to papillary muscle dysfunction or by mitral valve prolapse (Figure 4.5). Prolapse is defined by systolic movement of any part of either leaflet above the plane of the annulus in a long-axis view. Altogether about 5% of all people have some degree of mitral prolapse. Some patients with prolapse have abnormal collagen (e.g. Marfan or Ehlers–Danlos syndromes), but others in whom there is minor 'technical' prolapse are effectively normal. Thus minor echocardiographic prolapse must not automatically be assumed to be the cause of non-specific symptoms. Antibiotic prophylaxis is usually recommended only if there is more than trivial mitral regurgitation in association with prolapse. However, this question is still debated periodically. Other causes of mitral regurgitation include rheumatic disease and endocarditis (Figure 4.6).

Murmurs as a result of intracardiac shunts in adults are most frequently caused by a secundum atrial septal defect (Figure 4.7). Ventricular septal defects are the most common congenital anomalies in children and, since a membranous defect frequently fails to close, these may also be found in adults (Figure 4.8). A patent ductus arteriosus is occasionally diagnosed for the first time in an adult.

Quantification of valve disease
Aortic stenosis
The mobility of the aortic cusps on the two-dimensional or M-mode scans gives an approximate guide to severity, but Doppler ultrasound gives a far more accurate assessment. Using continuous wave Doppler, the velocity of blood flow across the valve is directly related to the degree of stenosis, because a pressure

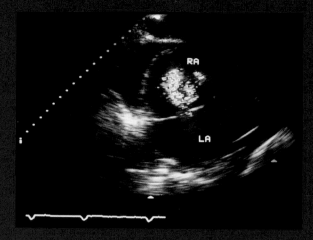

Figure 4.7 Secundum atrial septal defect. Subcostal view, clearly showing the origin of abnormal flow in the center of the atrial septum

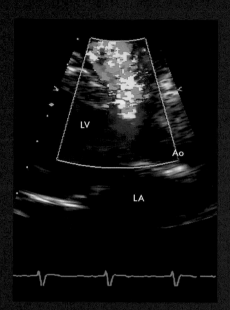

Figure 4.8
Perimembranous
ventricular septal
defect. Parasternal
long-axis view

Figure 4.9 Continuous wave recording from the apex in a patient with severe aortic stenosis. The signal has been traced giving an automated read-out of peak and mean pressure difference

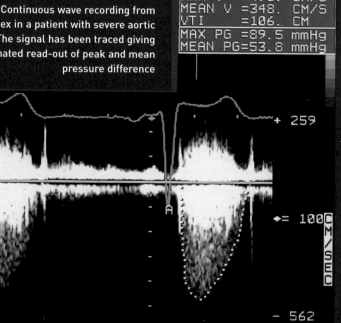

```
MAX V   =473.  CM/S
MEAN V  =348.  CM/S
VTI     =106.  CM
MAX PG  =89.5  mmHg
MEAN PG =53.8  mmHg
```

difference (loosely called a 'gradient') across a stenotic valve must be accompanied by an increase in the velocity of blood flow. These parameters are approximately related by the simplified **Bernoulli equation**: $\Delta P = 4v^2$ (where ΔP is pressure difference in mmHg and v is the velocity in m/s) as long as the peak velocity is $>3.0\,\text{m/s}$. For more mild aortic stenosis, this formula overestimates the pressure difference and no such estimate should usually be made. Mean pressure gradient is more accurate than peak gradient since it takes account of the whole rather than just the peak of the waveform. It is calculated automatically using online software by tracing round the waveform (Figure 4.9). The pressure differences estimated by Doppler echocardiography and cardiac catheterization are related but different (Figure 4.10) and should not be compared directly (Rijsterborgh and Roelendt, 1987).

The pressure difference across the aortic valve is dependent on cardiac output. If flow is high as a result of

Figure 4.10 Doppler ultrasound estimates the true peak instantaneous difference in pressure between the left ventricle and aorta (- - - -). At catheterization, it is usual to pull the catheter back across the aortic valve giving a 'pull-back' or 'peak-to-peak' gradient (——). The latter is not a true physiologic pressure difference, as the peaks on the aortic and left ventricular pressure waveforms do not occur simultaneously

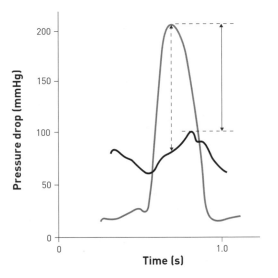

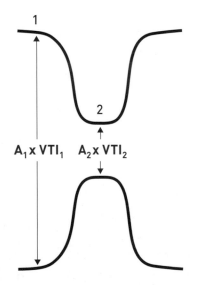

Figure 4.11 The principle of the continuity equation. The stroke volume at point 1 (subaortic level) must be the same as at point 2 (aortic valve level). Therefore the cross-sectional area at 1 x stroke distance at 1 must equal area at 2 x stroke distance at 2. By rearrangement: effective orifice area of the aortic valve is cross-sectional area of the subaortic region x subaortic stroke distance/aortic stroke distance. Subaortic velocity is recorded using pulsed Doppler with the sample in the left ventricular outflow tract; transaortic velocity is recorded using continuous wave Doppler

Table 4.2 Criteria for grading aortic stenosis		
	Mild stenosis	Severe stenosis
Peak velocity (m/s)	<3.0	>4.0
Peak gradient (mmHg)	<35	>65
Mean gradient (mmHg)	<20	>40
Effective orifice area (cm^2)	>1.2	<0.8

N.B. Intermediate values may either represent moderate disease or, if left ventricular function is impaired, may represent severe disease. This distinction may require referral for a specialist opinion

anemia or fever, the pressure difference will be elevated. Conversely, in a patient with heart failure, the pressure difference may be low. In such patients it is necessary to correct for the effect of flow and this is most frequently done with the **continuity equation**. This is based on the law of conservation of mass (Figure 4.11) and allows an estimated 'effective' orifice area to be calculated (Table 4.2). This is a hydraulic area and is different from and usually smaller than the anatomic orifice area. The normal adult anatomic area is 2.5–3.5 cm^2.

Because of the square relationship between pressure and velocity, small errors in velocity measurement or small changes as a result of varying left ventricular function can lead to misclassification of grade. Thus a peak instantaneous velocity of 3.5 m/s equates with a moderate pressure difference of about 50 mmHg, whilst a velocity of 4.5 m/s equates with a severe pressure difference of 80 mmHg. Furthermore, the significance of a pressure difference varies between individuals, depending largely on its effect on the left ventricle. Some patients with apparently moderate stenosis on hemodynamic criteria may become symptomatic and require operation, whilst others with high pressure differences may remain asymptomatic and be treated conservatively with relative safety.

Aortic regurgitation

Estimating the severity of regurgitation is more difficult than for aortic stenosis, and a balanced judgement must be made using a number of echocardiographic methods (Table 4.3) as well as the clinical examination. In general, Doppler is good for the diagnosis of severe

Table 4.3 Guideline thresholds for severe aortic regurgitation	
Continuous wave pressure half-time	<400 ms
Continuous wave slope	>3.0 m/s^2
Color flow height as proportion of LVOT height	>60%
Diastolic flow reversal beyond the aortic arch	present
Dilated volume loaded left ventricle	present

LVOT, left ventricular outflow tract

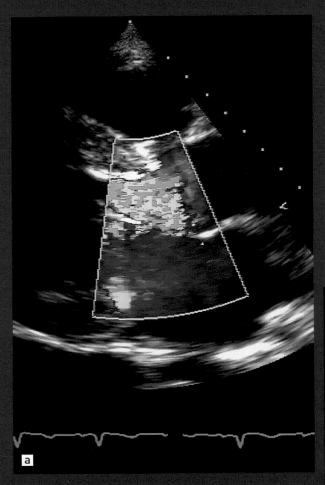

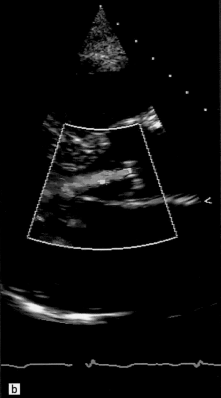

Figure 4.12 Aortic regurgitation on color flow mapping. The size of the defect in the valve is related to the size of the base of the jet. A convenient measure is the height of the jet expressed as a percentage of the height of the subaortic outflow tract measured about 0.5 cm below the valve. Severe regurgitation is shown by a ratio greater than 60%. In (a) the jet fills the whole of the outflow tract; (b) shows mild regurgitation

aortic regurgitation but cannot reliably differentiate mild from moderate regurgitation. Severity of regurgitation is related to the area of failed valvar apposition (the 'regurgitant orifice'), the pressure difference across the valve in diastole, and various hemodynamic factors such as the heart rate and the ability of the left ventricle to expand during diastole. The size of the regurgitant orifice is related to the height of the jet on color flow mapping (Figure 4.12). Severe regurgitation is likely if the jet occupies 60% or more of the full height of the left ventricular outflow tract. In severe aortic regurgitation, the pressure difference across the valve falls quickly and this shows as a steep deceleration slope on the continuous waveform (Figure 4.13). In severe aortic regurgitation, there is flow reversal lasting throughout diastole visible in the ascending aorta and beyond the arch.

Mitral stenosis

The mobility of the leaflet tips and the width of the color flow map through the valve give approximate guides to severity, but the area of the orifice can be measured directly in the two-dimensional short-axis view (Table 4.4). The orifice may be highly irregular and the reverberation from collagenous thickening or calcium deposits may

make it impossible to trace the orifice accurately. The Doppler recording of flow across the valve gives a direct hemodynamic assessment (Figure 4.14). For historical reasons, the rate of fall of the velocity signal is usually expressed as the pressure half-time rather than the slope. The pressure half-time is the time taken for the peak gradient to fall by half. Because of the square relationship between pressure and velocity, the pressure half-time becomes the time for peak velocity to fall to $1/\sqrt{2}$ of its original value ($1/\sqrt{2} = 0.7$). Pressure half-time is inversely related to orifice area by an empirical orifice area formula:

$$\text{Mitral orifice area (cm}^2) = 220/\text{pressure half-time}$$

This formula should not be applied if the pressure half-time is shorter than 150 ms, because in mild stenosis the half-time is significantly related to the diastolic behavior of the left atrium and ventricle. Even in moderate or severe mitral stenosis, the pressure half-time cannot produce a precise 'gold standard' orifice area. However, it is one of many useful guides to severity, which also include the

Table 4.4 Guideline criteria of severe stenosis	
Measured orifice area (cm²)	< 1.0
Mean gradient (mmHg)	> 10
Pressure half-time (ms)	> 200

Figure 4.13 The continuous wave signal in aortic regurgitation. In severe aortic regurgitation the pressure difference across the valve falls rapidly and the deceleration slope of the Doppler signal is correspondingly steep (**arrows**) (over 3 m/s^2)

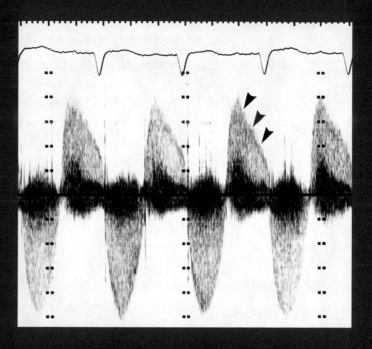

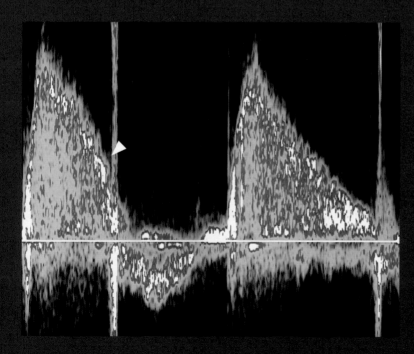

Figure 4.14 Mitral stenosis. On this continuous wave Doppler recording, velocities are raised throughout diastole, but are highly dependent on the length of the cycle. End-diastolic velocity is almost normal on the second complex but it is 1.6 m/s on the first (**arrow**)

speed of left ventricular filling and the pulmonary artery pressure.

The pulmonary artery pressure may be estimated from the transtricuspid pressure difference calculated from the tricuspid regurgitation jet using the Bernoulli equation added to an estimate of right atrial pressure. This is most accurately obtained from an assessment of the diameter of the inferior vena cava and its degree of collapse during inspiration.

The echocardiographer should then assess whether a valve is suitable for balloon valvotomy. This is a highly specialized judgement, which must be checked by transesophageal echocardiography, but in general a valve is suitable if there is significant mitral stenosis with:

- Mobile and unthickened anterior leaflet base

- No severe thickening of the chordae

- No commissural calcium

- No more than mild mitral regurgitation

- No visible left atrial thrombus.

Mitral regurgitation

The regurgitant fraction depends mainly on the size of the regurgitant orifice,

---

Table 4.5 Criteria of severe mitral regurgitation

- Color signal broad with prominent acceleration in the left ventricle
- Dense signal on continuous wave Doppler
- Systolic flow reversal in the pulmonary veins
- Volume overload of the left ventricle (e.g. fractional shortening >40%)
- Raised pulmonary artery pressure (usually systolic 25–50 mmHg)

---

the length of time it remains open, the systolic pressure difference across the valve, and the distensibility of the left atrium. With continuous wave Doppler, the density of the signal, in comparison to forward flow, provides an approximate guide to severity (Figure 4.15). The greater the regurgitant fraction, the more red cells there are to scatter ultrasound and therefore the more dense the signal. The area of the color flow map is strongly dependent on the instrument settings and the type of echo machine used. However, a jet area < 4 cm² strongly suggests mild and an area > 8 cm² strongly suggests severe regurgitation (Spain *et al.*, 1989) (Figure 4.16). However, the regurgitant color signal also consists of a region of flow acceleration in the left ventricle and a neck as the flow passes through the mitral valve. These are not susceptible to modification by hemodynamic events within the left atrium and are more reliable measures of grade (Table 4.5). A neck wider than 0.6 cm usually indicates severe regurgitation. The region of flow acceleration in the left ventricle

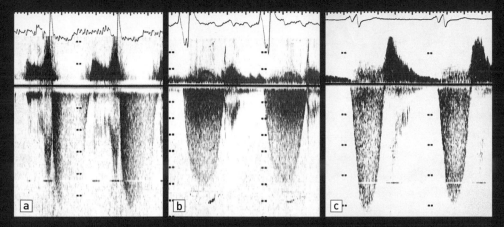

Figure 4.15 Mitral regurgitation continuous wave Doppler recording: (a) shows the low-intensity jet of mild regurgitation, (b) a medium jet, and (c) the dense jet of severe regurgitation

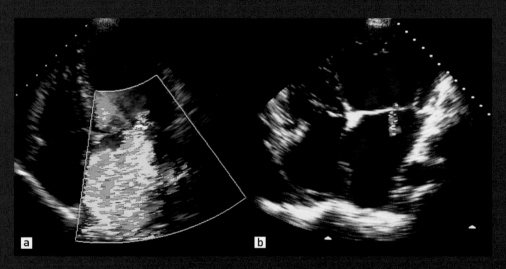

Figure 4.16 Mitral regurgitation color flow map. In severe regurgitation (a) the signal is wide with a large area whilst in mild regurgitation (b), it is narrow and has a small area

Figure 4.17 Vegetation. The patient had rheumatic mitral valve disease and presented with multiple transient ischemic attacks. There is an echogenic mass attached to the tip of the mitral valve prolapsing between the left atrium (left) and left ventricle (right)

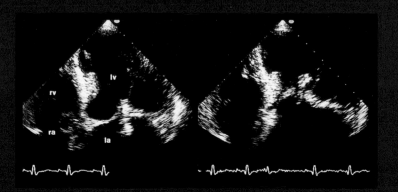

is directly related to the grade of regurgitation: small or absent in mild regurgitation and large in severe. Pulmonary flow patterns give another measure of grade of mitral regurgitation. In moderate regurgitation systolic forward flow may be blunted and in severe regurgitation, there is progressive systolic flow reversal. Indirect signs of regurgitation include a large and hyper-dynamic left ventricle and moderately raised pulmonary artery pressure.

Shunts

The size of the shunt in the presence of an atrial or ventricular septal defect can be estimated from the ratio of the pulmonary-to-aortic stroke volume.

Which murmurs do not need echocardiography?

Benign systolic flow murmurs or the murmur of mild aortic valve thickening do not need echocardiography. These are frequent in high flow states, anemia, fever, pregnancy and anxiety. They have the following characteristics:

- Short
- Soft or moderate in amplitude
- Ejection character
- Normal second heart sound
- May be louder on inspiration or lying.

Suspected endocarditis

The diagnosis is initially suspected on clinical grounds, usually by the presence of fever, an organism known to cause endocarditis, a new murmur or complications including embolic stroke, anemia, nail-fold infarcts and glomerulonephritis. The echocardiographic signs of endocarditis are:

- Vegetation
- Valve destruction
- Local complications (abscess, fistula, perforation, prosthetic valve dehiscence).

The diagnosis of endocarditis is aided by the Duke criteria (Table 4.6). Care is needed because echocardiography appears as both a major and minor criterion. A 'classical' vegetation is pedunculated, of low or intermediate echogenicity and moves out of phase with the valve to which it is attached (Figure 4.17). However, vegetations may sometimes be smaller, and hard to differentiate from the other causes of a mass attached to a valve: calcific degeneration, myxomatous degeneration, a cuspal tear, redundant chordae or a fibroelastoma. Minor thickening of a valve is common in the elderly and should not be overinterpreted as a major criterion.

For these reasons, echocardiography should not be part of a routine fever screen, but should usually be requested only if there is at least a moderate

Table 4.6 Duke criteria for endocarditis (either two major, or one major and three minor, or five minor criteria)

Major
- Persistently positive blood cultures with an organism known to cause endocarditis
- Echocardiographically definite vegetation or abscess or new prosthetic dehiscence or new native regurgitation

Minor
- Predisposing heart condition or intravenous drug use
- Fever
- Vascular phenomena: arterial emboli, septic pulmonary infarcts, intracranial hemorrhage, mycotic aneurysm, conjunctival hemorrhage
- Immunologic: glomerulonephritis
- Echocardiogram consistent with vegetation
- Positive blood culture, but not meeting major criterion

Reference: Durack DT, Lukes AS, Bright DK. New criteria for diagnosis of infective endocarditis: utilization of specific echocardiographic findings. Duke Endocarditis Service. *Am J Med* 1994;96:200–9

suspicion of disease. For example, a fever and ejection systolic murmur alone do not constitute sufficient evidence of endocarditis, since the murmur could be a result of high flow.

Which patients should be referred to a cardiologist?

The following groups are the minimum that should be referred for specialist advice:

- Suspected endocarditis
- Any symptomatic patient, since the presence of symptoms is a criterion for surgery in all types of valve disease

- Severe disease even in the absence of symptoms. Although surgery may not usually be performed in patients with severe aortic stenosis in the absence of symptoms there remains a small risk of sudden death and surgery may still be performed prophylactically. Similarly, in mitral stenosis where the left ventricle is protected by being downstream from the valve lesion, it is uncommon to operate in the absence of symptoms. However, the right ventricle may fail as a result of pulmonary hypertension and symptoms then diminish. The development of early right ventricular dysfunction on echocardiography is a warning sign arguing for prophylactic surgery

- Moderate aortic or mitral regurgitation. The timing of surgery for patients with severe regurgitant lesions is often difficult. There is the danger of leaving this so late that irreversible left ventricular damage supervenes. Furthermore, because the assessment of regurgitation is less precise than for stenotic lesions, it is safer to refer patients even with apparently moderate disease

- Any suggestion of impaired left ventricular systolic function. If the left ventricle is impaired, the severity of aortic stenosis may be underestimated. Furthermore, a reduction in measures of left ventricular systolic function represents a criterion for operating in aortic stenosis and both aortic and mitral regurgitation.

References

Lindner JR, Case RA, Dent JM, *et al.* Diagnostic value of echocardiography in suspected endocarditis. An evaluation based on the pretest probability of disease. *Circulation* 1996;**93**:730–6

Lindroos M, Kupari M, Heikkilä J, Tilvis R. Prevalence of aortic valve abnormalities in the elderly: an echocardiographic study of a random population sample. *J Am Coll Cardiol* 1993;**21**:1220–5

Rijsterborgh H, Roelendt J. Doppler assessment of aortic stenosis: Bernoulli revisited. *Ultrasound Med Biol* 1987;**13**:241–8

Spain MG, Smith MD, Grayburn PA, *et al.* Quantitative assessment of mitral regurgitation by Doppler color flow imaging: angiographic and hemodynamic correlations. *J Am Coll Cardiol* 1989;**13**:585–90

Further reading

Bonow RO, Carabello B, de Leon AC, *et al.* ACC/AHA guidelines for the management of patients with valvular heart disease. Executive Summary. *J Heart Valve Dis* 1998;**7**:672–707, *Circulation* 1998:**98**:1949–84

Oho CM. *Valvular Heart Disease*. Philadelphia: WB Saunders, 1999

Chapter 5

Hypertension

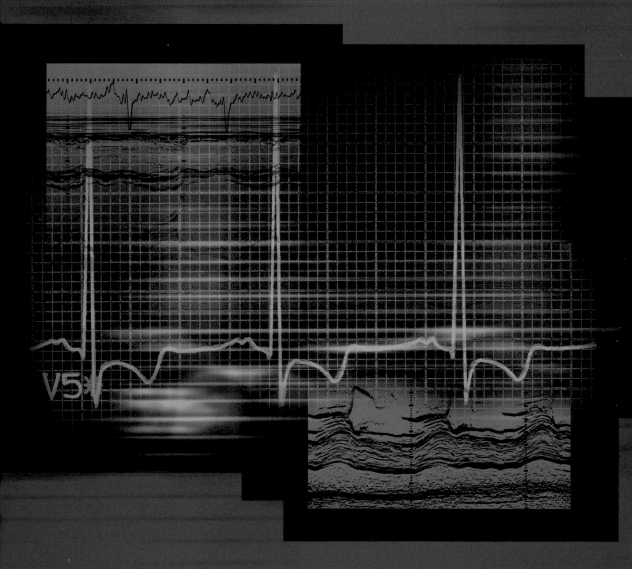

Left ventricular hypertrophy is an important risk factor for both myocardial infarction and sudden death, equivalent in impact to the presence of multivessel coronary disease (Liao *et al.*, 1995). The relative risk for all-cause mortality for every 50 g/m (indexed to height) increase in mass is 1.5 in men and 2.0 in women (Levy *et al.*, 1990). Left ventricular hypertrophy can therefore be used as an indication for treatment in patients with borderline hypertension (Table 5.1). Patients with unequivocal hypertension need not have echocardiography since the decision to treat is usually based on the level of blood pressure alone (Table 5.1). However, in young subjects, echocardiography should also be used to screen for coarctation.

Electrocardiographic hypertrophy is diagnosed if QRS voltages are high or if the strain pattern is present. Voltage criteria (e.g. R in V5 plus S in V2 > 35 mm) are non-specific since they may be seen in slim normal subjects. The strain pattern (Figure 5.1) consists of ST segment depression and T wave inversion in V5 and V6. This is highly specific for left ventricular hyper-trophy and is associated with a 7–9 times increased risk of heart failure in hypertensive patients. However, it is also insensitive. Overall, echocardiography is 5–10 times more sensitive at detecting left ventricular hypertrophy (Hammond *et al.*, 1988). An electrocardiogram is therefore not a viable alternative to echocardiography.

Left ventricular hypertrophy is usually diagnosed by the presence of absolute septal thickening; this is an insensitive way of making the diagnosis (Figure 5.2). An estimate of left ventricular (LV) mass (in g) should be obtained, for example using the Devereux formula based on septal (S) and posterior (PW) wall thickness in diastole, as well as left ventricular diastolic diameter (LVDD) (Devereux and Reicheck, 1977):

$$LV\ mass = 1.04\,[(S + PW + LVDD)^3 - LVDD^3] - 13.6$$

This should then be indexed to body habitus, for example to body surface

Table 5.1 Indications for echocardiography

Indicated
- Borderline hypertension/suspected white-coat/imperfect control
- If finding left ventricular hypertrophy will affect the decision to start or modify therapy
- Follow-up assessment in patients with left ventricular dysfunction

Not indicated
- Re-evaluation of asymptomatic patients
- Patients in whom the decision to treat has already been made

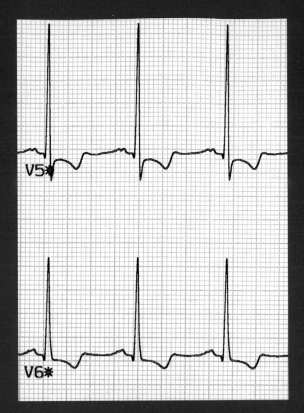

Figure 5.1 Electrocardiogram in left ventricular hypertrophy. There is ST segment depression and T wave inversion or left ventricular 'strain'

Figure 5.2 Echocardiogram in left ventricular hypertrophy. In (a) is an M-mode recording in a normal subject; (b) is from a patient with hypertension secondary to chronic renal failure

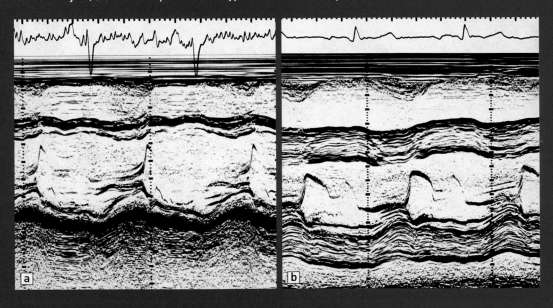

area (BSA). Well-accepted criteria for hypertrophy are left ventricular mass $> 134\,\mathrm{g/m^2}$ in men and $> 110\,\mathrm{g/m^2}$ in women (Hammond *et al.*, 1988). At the same time, left ventricular geometry should be assessed. By the law of Laplace, left ventricular wall stress (S) is directly proportional to intracavitary pressure (P) and chamber radius (R) and is inversely proportional to wall thickness (Th) ($S = P.R / Th$). Left ventricular hypertrophy tends to reduce wall stress by increasing wall thickness and reducing cavity size. However, the relationship between left ventricular mass, cavity size and pressure is not fixed. Three different geometric responses can be defined by the relative wall

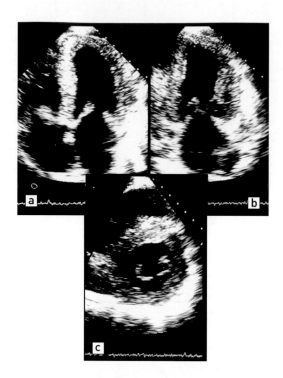

Figure 5.3 Two-dimensional image for calculation of left ventricular mass. The four-chamber and two-chamber apical views (**a** and **b**) are used for determination of major long-axis dimensions. Cross-sectional myocardial area is calculated from planimetry of epicardial borders in the short-axis view at the papillary muscle level (**c**)

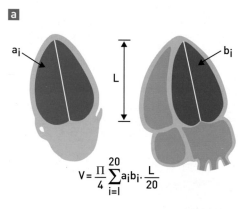

$$V = \frac{\Pi}{4} \sum_{i=1}^{20} a_i b_i \cdot \frac{L}{20}$$

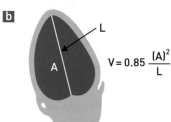

$$V = 0.85 \frac{(A)^2}{L}$$

Figure 5.4 Calculation of left ventricular volume. (**a**) Method of disks. Calculation of volume is from summation of areas from diameters a_i and b_i of disks of equal height; apportioned by dividing left ventricular longest length (L) into equal sections. (**b**) Single plane area length. Useful if only one apical view is obtainable. A, area of left ventricular cavity; L, length of left ventricular cavity. Myocardial volume is then multiplied by 1.04 to calculate left ventricular mass.

Adapted with permission from Schiller NB, Shah PM, Crawford M, *et al. J Am Soc Echocardiogr* 1989;2:358–67

thickness ratio (RWT ratio), which is the thickness of the posterior wall divided by left ventricular radius in diastole:

- Concentric hypertrophy defined by increased left ventricular mass and a high relative wall thickness ratio (>0.45)

- Eccentric hypertrophy defined by increased left ventricular mass and normal relative wall thickness ratio (<0.45)

- Concentric remodeling defined by normal left ventricular mass with a high wall thickness ratio (>0.45). Concentric remodeling is associated with an increased risk of morbid events (2.39 per 100 patient years) compared with normal geometry (1.12 per 100 patient years) (Verdecchia et al., 1995).

Left ventricular mass can also be calculated by two-dimensional echocardiography using either the area/length or the truncated ellipsoid methods (Figures 5.3 and 5.4). Both correlate well with anatomic left ventricular mass provided that care is taken to avoid foreshortening the left ventricular cavity. Correlations are better than by M-mode, especially in hearts with abnormal geometry, and reproducibility is also better (Collins et al., 1989). Despite this, these two-dimensional methods are seldom used, mainly because they are more time-consuming and partly because so much experience with M-mode already exists. Three-dimensional techniques show promise but remain research-based.

What technique should be used for research studies?

There is potentially major intra- and interobserver variability in M-mode measurements which can be minimized by averaging at least 3–5 cycles. In the PRESERVE trial (Prospective Randomized Enalapril Study Evaluating Regression of Ventricular Enlargement), the between-study standard deviation in left ventricular mass was only $6\,g/m^2$ (Devereux et al., 1996). However, standard deviations may sometimes be as high as 30 g (Goltdiener et al., 1995) which is of the same magnitude as expected changes in left ventricular mass. This means that M-mode measurements should rarely be used for quantifying a change in left ventricular mass over serial studies in small populations. In trials with a large population of more than several hundred patients, echocardiography remains a suitable technique, and a number of recent studies of left ventricular hypertrophy have used this method (Dahlöf et al., 1997; Devereux et al., 1996; Gosse et al., 1998; Gosse et al., 2000).

Nuclear magnetic resonance imaging has superior image quality compared to echocardiography and yields truly tomographic images with little reliance on geometric assumptions. Magnetic resonance imaging has been validated against anatomic mass in cadaver hearts and in dogs' hearts compared to subsequent post-mortem assessment. It is accurate in assessing asymmetric hearts, for example in dogs with experimentally induced myocardial infarction or in humans with hypertrophic cardiomyopathy (Soler *et al.*, 1999). The standard error in estimating left ventricular mass is about one-third of that of echocardiography so that magnetic resonance imaging is more accurate for serial estimates of left ventricular mass (Boudoulas, 1997).

References

Boudoulas H. Determination of left ventricular mass in clinical practice. *J Heart Valve Dis* 1997;**6**:222–7

Collins HW, Kronenberg MW, Byrd BF. Reproducibility of left ventricular mass measurements by two-dimensional and M-mode echocardiography. *J Am Coll Cardiol* 1989;**14**:672–6

Dahlöf B. Effect of angiotensin II blockade on cardiac hypertrophy and remodelling: a review. *J Hum Hypertens* 1995;**9**(Suppl 5):537–44

Dahlöf B, Devereux R, de Faire U, *et al.* The losartan intervention for endpoint reduction (LIFE) in hypertension study: rationale, design and methods. The LIFE study group. *Am J Hypertens* 1997;**10**:705–13

Devereux RB, Dahlof B, Levy D, Pfeffer MA. Comparison of enalapril versus nifedipine to decrease left ventricular hypertrophy in systemic hypertension (the PRESERVE trial). *Am J Cardiol* 1996;**78**:61–5

Devereux RB, Reicheck NR. Echocardiographic determination of left ventricular mass in man: anatomic validation of the method. *Circulation* 1977;**55**:613–18

Gosse P, Guez D, Gueret P, *et al.* Centralized echocardiogram quality control in a multicenter study of regression of left ventricular hypertophy in hypertension. *J Hypertens* 1998;**16**:531–5

Gosse P, Sheridan DJ, Zannad F, *et al.* Regression of left ventricular hypertrophy in hypertensive patients treated with indapamide SR 1.5mg versus enalapril 20mg: the LIVE study. *J Hypertens* 2000;**18**:1465–75

Gottdiener JS, Livengood SV, Meyer PS, Chase GA. Should echocardiography be performed to assess effects of antihypertensive therapy? Test-retest reliability of echocardiography for measurement of left ventricular mass and function. *J Am Coll Cardiol* 1995;**25**:424–30

Hammond IW, Devereux RB, Alderman MH, *et al.* Prevalence and correlates of echocardiographic left ventricular hypertrophy among employed patients with uncomplicated hypertension. *J Am Coll Cardiol* 1988;**7**:639–50

Levy D, Garrison RJ, Savage DD, *et al.* Prognostic implications of echocardiographically determined left ventricular mass in the Framingham Heart Study. *N Engl J Med* 1990;**322**:1561–6

Liao Y, Cooper RS, McGee DL, *et al.* The relative effects of left ventricular hypertrophy, coronary artery disease and left ventricular dysfunction on survival among black adults. *JAMA* 1995;**273**:1592–7

Soler R, Rodriguez E, Marini M. Left ventricular mass in hypertrophic cardiomyopathy: assessment by three-dimensional and geometric MR methods. *J Comput Assist Tomogr* 1999;**23**:577–82

Verdecchia P, Schillaci G, Borgioni C, *et al.* Adverse prognostic significance of concentric remodeling of the left ventricle in hypertensive patients with normal left ventricular mass. *J Am Coll Cardiol* 1995;**25**:871–8

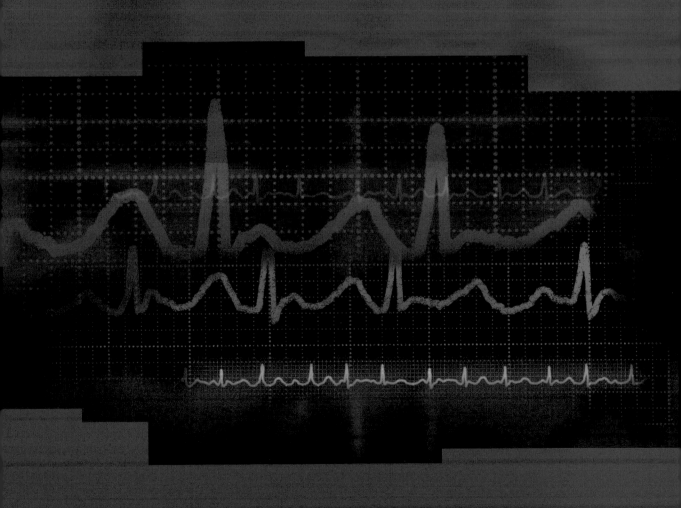

Chapter 6

Arrhythmias

Table 6.1 Echocardiography in arrhythmias and syncope

Indicated

- Clinical suspicion of structural disease e.g. ventricular tachycardia or atrial fibrillation aged <60 or abnormal cardiovascular examination
- Family history of a transmissible disease e.g. tuberous sclerosis, hypertrophic cardiomyopathy
- Prior to radiofrequency ablation
- Before cardioversion (transesophageal echocardiography; see p.74)
- Exertional syncope or syncope in high-risk occupation e.g. pilot
- Arrhythmia requiring treatment (Class IIa indication)

Not indicated

- Palpitation with no abnormal signs or corresponding arrhythmia
- Ventricular premature complexes and no clinical suspicion of heart disease
- Before cardioversion if on long-term anticoagulation, atrial fibrillation of <48 hours' duration and no structural heart disease, emergency cardioversion necessary
- Classic neurogenic syncope or syncope with no evidence of heart disease on history or exam
- After radiofrequency ablation in the absence of complications

Echocardiography is indicated if there is suspicion of underlying cardiac disease, based on the presence of atrial fibrillation, ventricular tachycardia or significant abnormalities on clinical examination or the electrocardiogram. It can help define thromboembolic risk in atrial fibrillation and is also indicated as a prelude to cardioversion (Table 6.1). Echocardiography is not indicated for palpitation or ventricular premature complexes alone.

Atrial fibrillation (Figure 6.1) is not a complete diagnosis, and a number of underlying causes need to be looked for and excluded, including ischemic heart disease, cardiomyopathy, hypertension, mitral valve disease, and thyrotoxicosis. Once done, and provided the patient is under 60 years of age, a diagnosis of lone atrial fibrillation can be made. For the purposes of anticoagulation treatment, there are effectively three categories of atrial fibrillation:

- rheumatic
- non-rheumatic
- lone atrial fibrillation.

Lone atrial fibrillation is a benign condition which does not carry the risk of thromboembolism so that anticoagulation with warfarin is not required. The need for warfarin is clear in the presence of rheumatic disease. For non-rheumatic disease, there may be uncertainty over whether the benefit of anticoagulation outweighs the risk of bleeding. The benefit is a fall in the risk of stroke overall by 60% (Boston Area

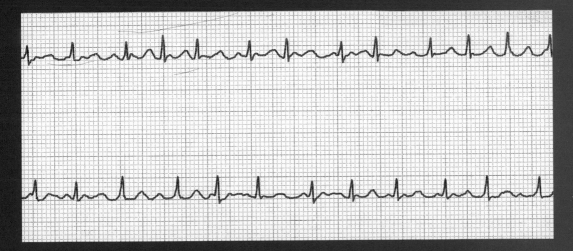

Figure 6.1 An electrocardiogram showing atrial fibrillation

Table 6.2 The annual risk of stroke rises if a patient has left atrial (LA) enlargement or left ventricular (LV) dysfunction	
Findings	**Annual risk (%)**
Sinus rhythm (normal heart)	0.3
Lone AF	0.5
AF + normal echo	1.5
AF + LA >2.5 cm/m²	8.8
AF + global LV dysfunction	12.6
AF + LA >2.5 cm/m² and moderate LV dysfunction	20.00

AF, atrial fibrillation. Left atrial area was used. This is not a widely-applied measure but is intuitively sensible. **Reference:** Stroke Prevention in Atrial Fibrillation Study Group Investigators. *Ann Intern Med* 1992;116;6 –12

Anticoagulation Trial, 1990; Stroke Prevention in Atrial Fibrillation Study, 1992), while the risk of bleeding is variable (up to 5% per year). Most factors determining an increased risk of thrombo-embolism are clinical (diabetes, hypertension, heart failure, previous stroke or TIA, age over 75 years). However, echocardiography can sometimes be used to aid the decision whether to anticoagulate. There is some evidence that, with a normal echocardiogram, the risk of stroke is small, even with associated atrial fibrillation. However, this risk rises sharply if there is left atrial enlargement or left ventricular dysfunction (Table 6.2).

The role of transesophageal echocardiography before DC cardioversion remains under discussion. It is currently indicated (Klein *et al.*, 2001) if:

- atrial fibrillation is present for >48 hours and early cardioversion is desired

- atrial fibrillation is present for <48 hours but structural heart disease is present

- anticoagulation is contraindicated

- previous thromboembolic event or left atrial thrombus demonstrated.

References

Boston Area Anticoagulation Trial for Atrial Fibrillation Investigators. The effect of low dose warfarin in the risk of stroke in patients with nonrheumatic atrial fibrillation. *N Engl J Med* 1990;**323**:1505–11

Klein AL, Grimm RA, Murray RD, *et al.* Use of transesophageal echocardiography to guide cardioversion in patients with atrial fibrillation. *N Engl J Med* 2001;**344**:1411–20.

Klein AL, Murray RD, Grimm RA. Role of transesophageal echocardiography-guided cardioversion of patients with atrial fibrillation. *J Am Coll Cardiol* 2001;**37**:691–704

Stroke Prevention in Atrial Fibrillation Study Group Investigators. Predictors of thromboembolism in atrial fibrillation. II. Echocardiographic features of patients at risk. *Ann Intern Med* 1992;**116**:6–12

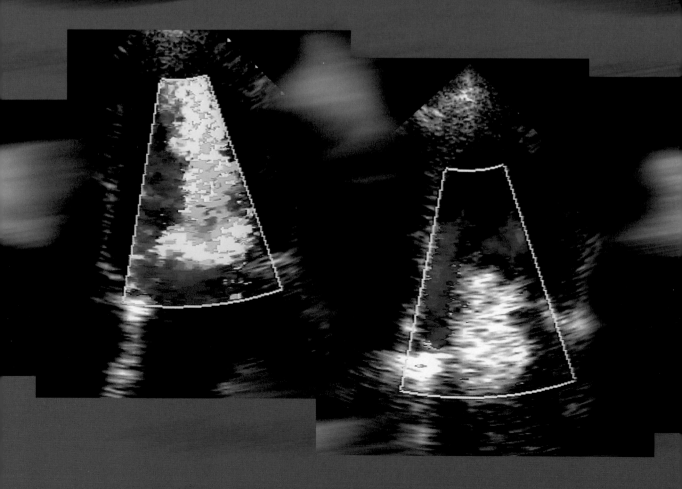

Chapter 7

Stroke, transient ischemic attack and peripheral emboli

The main purpose of echocardiography is to detect or confirm:

- a diagnosis known to be associated with a risk of thromboembolism, such as left ventricular dilatation or mitral stenosis

- a direct source of emboli such as thrombus, myxoma or vegetation.

Of these, the presence of an underlying substrate for thromboembolism is the more important. Thus, the risk of thromboembolism is so high in the presence of mitral stenosis that it can be assumed to be the cause of cerebral infarction even in the absence of left atrial thrombus (which may be too small for detection or may already have embolized).

However, occasionally a direct source of emboli is discovered, usually a thrombus (Figure 7.1), and occasionally a myxoma (Figure 7.2). If there is a clinically obvious cause of stroke, echocardiography is still indicated since it may refine the diagnosis. An example is the detection of a ball thrombus (Figure 7.3) in a patient with mitral stenosis since this is an indication for urgent surgery.

In subjects aged under 50 years, it is generally accepted that a full study including transesophageal echocardiography should be performed even in the absence of clinical abnormalities. This is mainly to look for rare treatable causes of stroke such as occult left atrial myxoma, endocarditis or left atrial thrombus (Figure 7.4). Other abnormalities on

---

Table 7.1 Echocardiography in stroke, transient ischemic attack and peripheral emboli

Indicated
- Any patient with abrupt occlusion of a major peripheral or visceral artery (transesophageal echocardiography)
- Clinical evidence of relevant structural heart disease e.g. mitral stenosis
- Clinical suggestion of endocarditis, myxoma or aortic dissection
- Patients aged < 50 years* with cerebral infarction (transesophageal echocardiography)
- Patients aged > 50 years* without evidence of cerebrovascular disease or other obvious cause in whom the findings of echocardiography will change management (e.g. to start warfarin if a patent foramen ovale is found) (transesophageal echocardiography)
- Strong suggestion of cardiac emboli (e.g. peripheral and cerebral events) (transesophageal echocardiography)

Not indicated
- The results of echocardiography will not affect treatment
- Intrinsic cerebrovascular disease sufficient to cause the clinical event

* The American College of Cardiology/American Heart Association guidelines suggest a threshold age of 45 years, but 50 years is common clinical practice in Europe

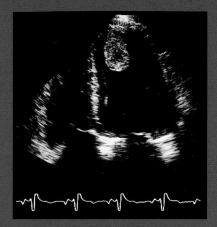

Figure 7.1 Left
ventricular thrombus

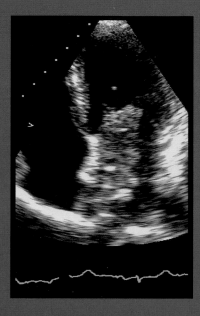

Figure 7.2 Left atrial
myxoma. There is a large
mass attached to the
atrial septum and
prolapsing through the
mitral valve during
diastole. Transthoracic
four-chamber view

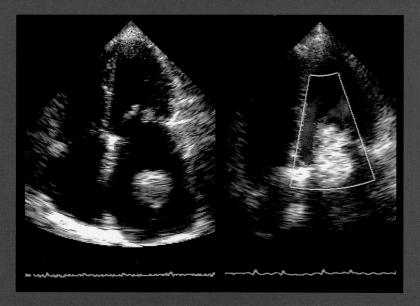

Figure 7.3 Ball thrombus
in a patient with mitral
stenosis. In systole (**left**),
the thrombus lies towards
the base of the greatly
enlarged left atrium; in
diastole (**right**) it enters
the mitral orifice, virtually
occluding forward flow

Figure 7.4 Left atrial appendage thrombus. The appendage contains a mass (arrowed) at its mouth. About 85% of left atrial thrombi develop in the appendage. They usually occur in the presence of general thromboembolic risk factors such as atrial fibrillation or mitral valve disease. However, rarely, they also occur in a patient with no structural disease in sinus rhythm

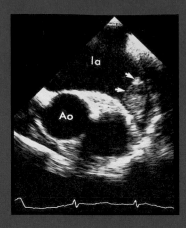

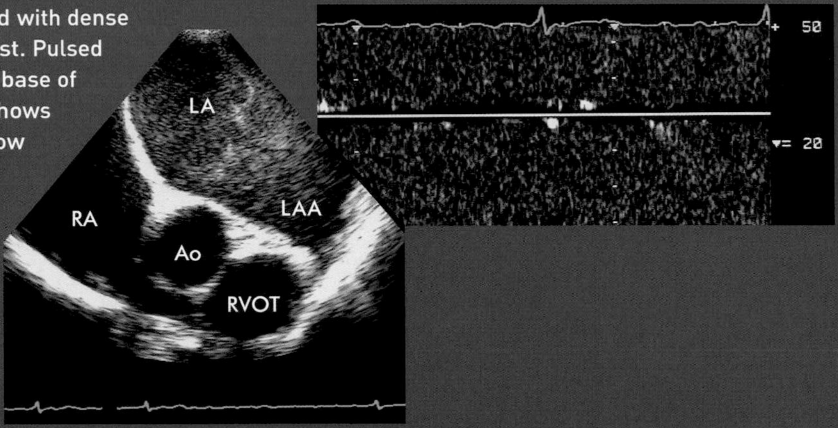

Figure 7.5 Left atrial spontaneous contrast. The left atrium and appendage are large and filled with dense spontaneous contrast. Pulsed Doppler recording at the base of the appendage shows virtually absent flow into and out of the appendage, indicating a high risk of thrombus formation. **LAA**, left atrial appendage; **RVOT**, right ventricular outflow tract

Figure 7.6 Transesophageal echocardiography after stroke. The patient was a young woman with severe asthma controlled by regular injections of methylprednisolone given via an indwelling subclavian line. She had a stroke followed by an embolism to the left leg. Echocardiography showed a thrombus attached to the right atrial part of the line (**a**) and contrast injection (**b**) showed passage of a small number of microbubbles (arrow) across a patent foramen ovale. After 1 week of intravenous heparin the mass had resolved (**c**)

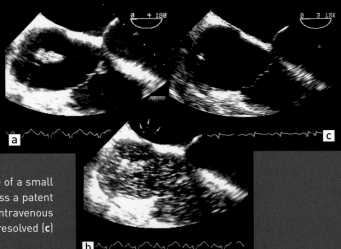

transesophageal echocardiography that may be relevant are left atrial spontaneous contrast (implying a higher than average risk of thromboembolism; Figure 7.5), patent foramen ovale (allowing the passage of venous thrombus from right to left heart; Figures 7.6 and 7.7) and aortic atheroma (Figure 7.8).

Echocardiography should also be considered in patients older than 50 if no other cause for the stroke is found or if there is a strong suggestion of a cardiac source for emboli (e.g. a combination of both peripheral and cerebral events or infarction in more than one territory).

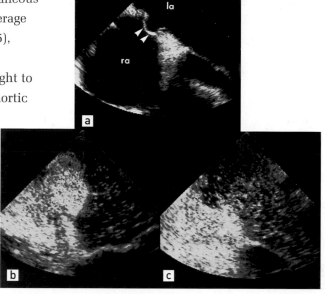

Figure 7.7 Atrial septal aneurysm and patent foramen ovale. An aneurysmal atrial septum (**a, arrows**) is found in about 15% after ischemic stroke compared with 3% of the general population. Of these about 75% are associated with a patent foramen ovale, in this case largely (**b, c**) defined by the passage of >20 microbubbles

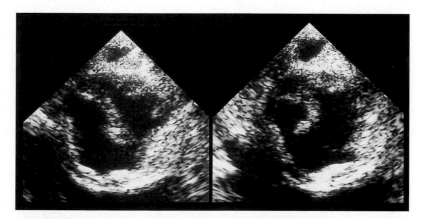

Figure 7.8 Aortic atheroma. These are transverse sections through the upper descending thoracic aorta showing a large, mobile, pedunculated mass of atheroma. Aortic atheroma is common. There is an association with peripheral emboli only if the atheroma is large (>5 mm in depth) or complex (mobile, pedunculated or ulcerated)

Further reading

Cerebral Embolism Task Force. Cardiogenic brain embolism. *Arch Neurol* 1989;**46**:727–43

Chambers J, de Belder M, Moore D. Echocardiography in stroke and transient ischaemic attack. *Heart* 1997;**78**(Suppl 1):2–6

Homma S, DiTullio MR. Cardiac sources of embolus: how to find it. *ACC Current J Rev* 2001;**10**:45–8

Schapiro LM, Westgate CJ, Shine K, Donaldson R. Is cardiac ultrasound mandatory in all patients with systemic emboli? *Br Med J* 1985;**291**:786–7

Chapter 8

Myocardial infarction

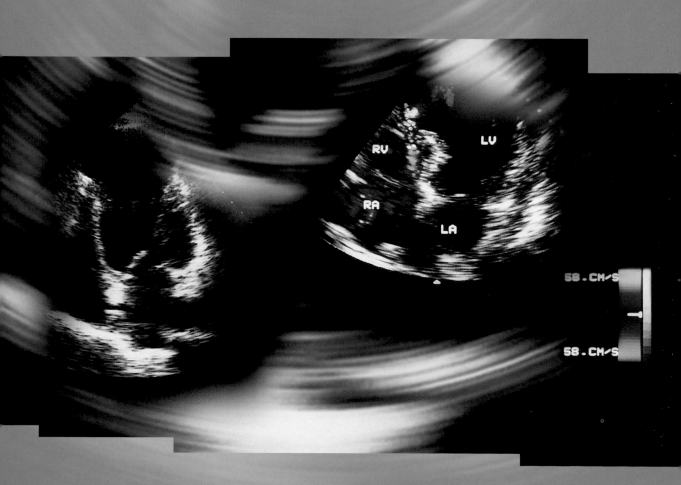

Echocardiography is occasionally indicated for the diagnosis of an acute coronary syndrome. A wall abnormality may be seen in the presence of a normal or equivocal electrocardiogram, especially in the presence of free wall infarction. Echocardiography is also indicated for the diagnosis of right ventricular infarction as suspected clinically by the presence of hypotension and a raised jugular venous pressure (Figure 8.1, Table 8.1).

Most centers will assess left ventricular function routinely, usually 3–5 days postinfarction, as a measure of the residual damage and also to refine whether to start or to stay on angiotensin converting enzyme (ACE) inhibitors. Regional and global systolic function must be assessed (see Chapter 3). Mitral regurgitation occurs commonly either as a result of papillary muscle dysfunction (elongation or splaying) or akinesis of the inferior wall (Figure 8.2).

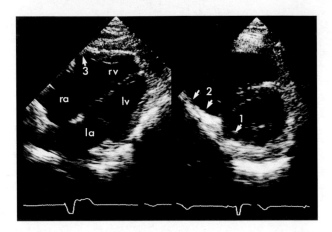

Figure 8.1 Right ventricular infarction. There is an infarct of the inferior wall of the left ventricle (**1**) with thinning and akinesis of the adjacent part of the right ventricle (**2**). The base of the right ventricular free wall is also affected (**3**)

Table 8.1 Echocardiography in chest pain (see also Table 1.3)

Indicated
- Diagnosis of ischemia if not possible using standard investigations and if the echocardiography can be performed soon after pain
- Suspicion of postinfarct complication (pansystolic murmur, cardiogenic shock)
- Postinfarction to assess left ventricular function if this will change management (e.g. starting angiotensin converting enzyme (ACE) inhibitor)
- Suspected aortic dissection (transesophageal echocardiography)
- Suspected right ventricular involvement

Not indicated
- Stable angina or pain thought to be non-cardiac
- Acute coronary syndrome already diagnosed by other criteria
- Routine re-evaluation in the absence of any change in clinical status

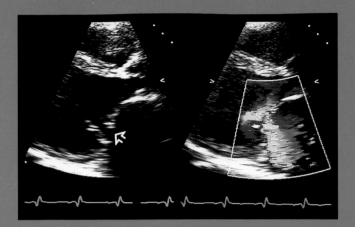

Figure 8.2 Mitral regurgitation following inferior infarction as a result of restriction of the posterior mitral leaflet. The akinetic inferobasal wall is unable to shorten during systole to allow the posterior leaflet to fall back into the orifice to be level with the anterior leaflet. The jet of regurgitation is directed posteriorly

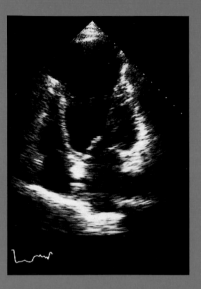

Figure 8.3 Left ventricular aneurysm. There is a large bulge with a wide neck at the apex of the left ventricle

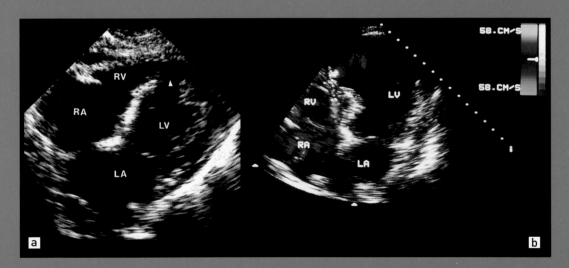

Figure 8.4 Ventricular septal rupture. An apical defect is shown (**arrow**) on a subcostal four-chamber view (**a**). In another patient (**b**) there is a bulge at the apex caused by the anterior infarct and the rupture is marked by a stream of blue on color flow mapping

A complication of infarction (Table 8.2) is an indication for immediate echocardiography as indicated by the development of heart failure or a pansystolic murmur.

Table 8.2 Complications after acute myocardial infarction

- Aneurysm (Figure 8.3)
- Pseudoaneurysm
- Ventricular septal rupture (Figure 8.4)
- Free wall rupture
- Papillary muscle rupture
- Thrombus

Stress echocardiography (see page 23) is useful for stratifying the risk of a subsequent coronary event and therefore for planning invasive investigation and intervention. In patients with signifi-cantly impaired left ventricular function, dobutamine stress echocardiography can identify viability in regions of abnormal wall motion. There is a higher mortality in patients with myocardial viability who are not revascularized than in those with no viability at all. However, there is an improved prognosis in those with viability who are revascularized (Lee *et al.,* 1994).

Further reading

D'Arcy B, Nanda NC. Two-dimensional echocardiographic features of right ventricular infarction. *Circulation* 1982;**65**:167–73

Jaarsma W, Visser CA, Eenige MJ, *et al.* Predictive value of two-dimensional echocardiographic and hemodynamic measurements on admission with acute myocardial infarction. *J Am Soc Echogr* 1988;**1**:187–93

Kono T, Sabbah HN, Rosman H, *et al.* Mechanism of functional mitral regurgitation during acute myocardial ischaemia. *J Am Coll Cardiol* 1992;**19**:1101–15

Lee KS, Marwick TH, Cook SA, *et al.* Prognosis of patients with left ventricular dysfunction with and without viable myocardium after myocardial infarction. Relative efficiency of medical therapy and revascularization. *Circulation* 1994;**90**:2687–94

Miyatake K, Okomoto M, Kinoshita N, *et al.* Doppler echocardiographic features of ventricular septal rupture in myocardial infarction. *J Am Coll Cardiol* 1985;**5**:182–7

Visser LA, Kan G, Meltger RS, *et al.* Incidence, timing and prognostic value of left ventricular aneurysm formation after myocardial infarction: a prospective serial echocardiographic study of 158 patients. *Am J Cardiol* 1986;**57**:729–32

Chapter 9

Pericardial disease

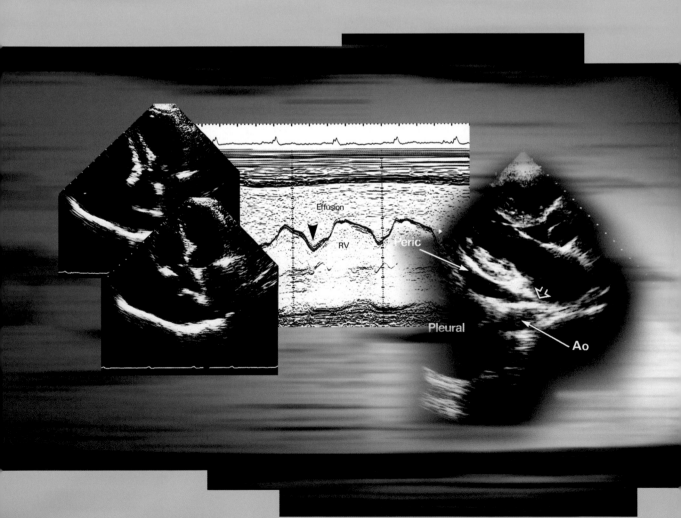

Echocardiography is not usually indicated in suspected pericarditis since the diagnosis relies on the history, the examination and the electrocardiogram. Pericardial fluid (Figure 9.1) is a non-specific finding in normal subjects or in the presence of hypoalbuminemia.

Table 9.1 Echocardiography in pericardial disease
Indicated
● Suspected effusion or constriction
● Large effusion to document early signs of tamponade
● Suspected pericardial bleed after trauma
● Echocardiography-guided pericardiocentesis
Not indicated
● Routine follow-up of a small effusion
● Follow-up studies in patients in whom management will not be affected by echocardiographic findings
● Friction rub after myocardial infarction or heart surgery
● Pericarditis in the absence of evidence of myocarditis or tamponade

However echocardiography becomes important if there is evidence either of myocarditis (e.g. loss of R wave on the electrocardiogram, a rise in levels of cardiac enzymes or pulmonary edema on the chest radiograph) or of tamponade (Table 9.1). The echocardiographic signs of tamponade in the presence of pericardial fluid are (Appleton *et al.*, 1987):

- Collapse of the right ventricle during diastole (Figure 9.2)

- A fall in left-sided velocities on inspiration, usually by >30%

- A dilated inferior vena cava which fails to collapse during inspiration (see also Figure 3.8).

Pericardial constriction should be suspected in the presence of a raised jugular venous pressure and normal left and right ventricular systolic function on echocardiography. The classical echocardiographic findings are (Appleton *et al.*, 1988; Borganelli & Byrd, 1990):

- Fast filling pattern on the transmitral pulsed recording (E deceleration <140 ms)

- Increased respiratory swing with a fall in E velocity >30% on inspiration (Figure 9.3)

- Increased flow reversal on expiration in the superior vena cava during atrial systole.

References

Appleton C, Hatle L, Popp R. Superior vena cava and hepatic vein Doppler echocardiography in healthy adults. *J Am Coll Cardiol* 1987;**10**:1032 9

Figure 9.1 Pericardial (Peric) and pleural effusions. These can be differentiated from the relative position of the descending thoracic aorta. The pericardial effusion finishes anterior (**arrow**) and the pleural effusion posterior to the descending aorta

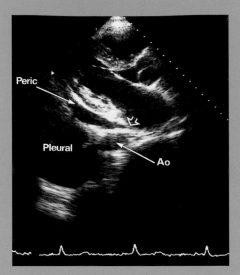

Figure 9.2 Pericardial tamponade. There is collapse of the whole of the free wall of the right ventricle throughout diastole (**arrow**)

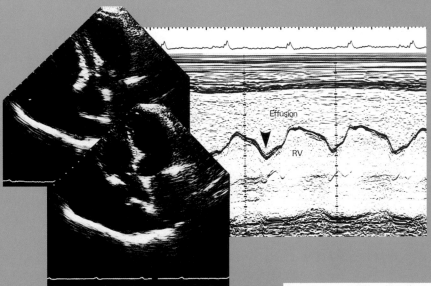

Figure 9.3 Pericardial constriction. There is thickening of the pericardium (**a**) although this is a non-specific and insensitive sign on echocardiography. The aortic signal disappears on inspiration (**arrow**) and the mitral E wave (**Ei**) is lower than on expiration (**Ee**) by >30%

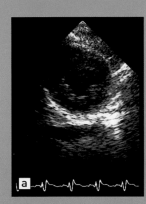

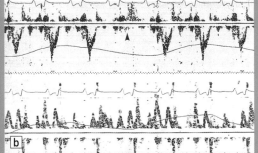

Appleton C, Hatle L, Popp R. Cardiac
tamponade and pericardial effusion:
respiratory variation in transvalvular flow
velocities studied by echocardiography.
J Am Coll Cardiol 1988;**11**:1020–33

Borganelli M, Byrd BF. Doppler echocardiography in pericardial disease. *Cardiol Clin*
1990;**8**:333–48

Oh JK, Hatle L, Seward JB. Diagnostic role
of Doppler echocardiography in constrictive
pericarditis. *J Am Coll Cardiol* 1994;**23**:154–62

Chapter 10

Aorta

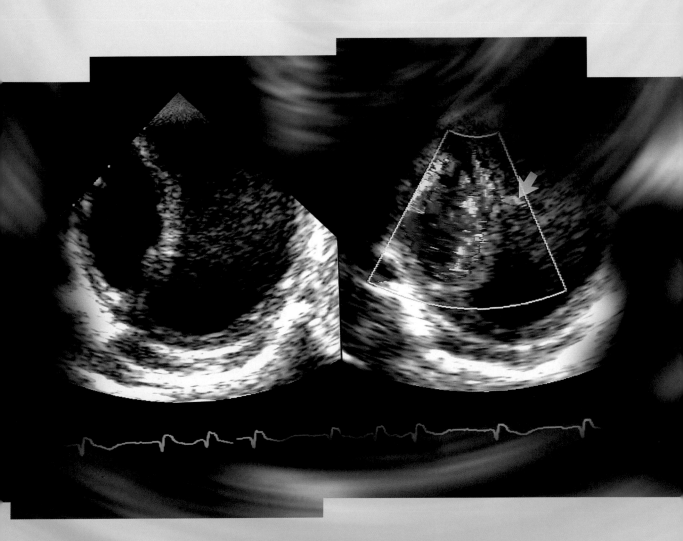

Echocardiography is used to detect aortic ectasia or aortic dissection. It is indicated if the chest radiograph is abnormal or there is a condition associated with dilatation (e.g. Marfan syndrome, bicuspid aortic valve) or if the history of acute chest pain suggests dissection (Table 10.1). The aorta must also be examined in patients with aortic regurgitation.

The diameter of the aorta should be measured at every important level, including the annulus, sinus of Valsalva, sinotubular junction, arch and descending thoracic and abdominal aorta (see also Figure 2.11). In the ascending aorta, the level of dilatation may be affected by the under-lying abnormality. In Marfan syndrome, the sinus of Valsalva typically becomes dilated (Figure 10.1) while in ectasia of old age or hypertension, the higher ascending aorta (Figure 10.2) becomes dilated. Surgery is often recommended if the diameter exceeds 5.0 cm in Marfan syndrome or 6.0 cm in the dilatation of old age or hypertension. However these thresholds vary in individual cases depending on the presence of symptoms, aortic regurgitation or the rate of progression of dilatation.

In suspected dissection transthoracic echocardiography detects a flap in 50% of cases of type A dissection (involving only the ascending aorta) (Figure 10.3) and about 30% of type B dissections (involving only the descending thoracic aorta). This may be enough to determine the need for surgery. Transesophageal echocardiography provides a higher resolution view, allowing the visualization of the:

- Flap
- Entry point
- Involvement of the head and neck vessels
- State of the aortic valve
- Presence of pericardial fluid and state of the left ventricle.

The sensitivity and specificity of transesophageal echocardiography and spiral computed tomography (CT) are similar for the diagnosis of dissection. In general if the clinical scenario is highly suggestive, transesophageal echocardiography can be done in the intensive therapy unit or even on the table as final proof. If, however, the diagnosis is uncertain, transesophageal echocardiography or CT can be done according to local expertise.

Table 10.1 Echocardiography in diseases of the aorta

Indicated
- Suspected aortic dissection or rupture (may also need transesophageal echocardiography)
- Widened mediastinum on the chest radiograph
- Serial studies if the ascending aorta is dilated
- Conditions associated with dilatation of the aorta e.g. Marfan syndrome

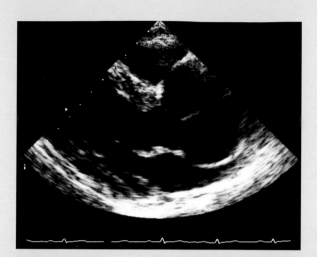

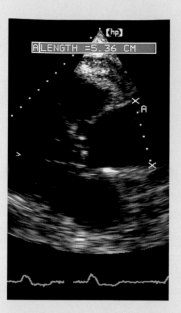

Figure 10.1 Annulo-aortic ectasia in Marfan syndrome. The annulus is 28 mm in diameter, the sinus of Valsalva is 58 mm and the sinotubular junction 50 mm. The normal sinotubular junction has a similar diameter to the annulus

Figure 10.2 Aortic ectasia. A parasternal long-axis view in a 79-year-old man. The annulus and sinus of Valsalva are normal, but the ascending aorta is dilated to 54 mm

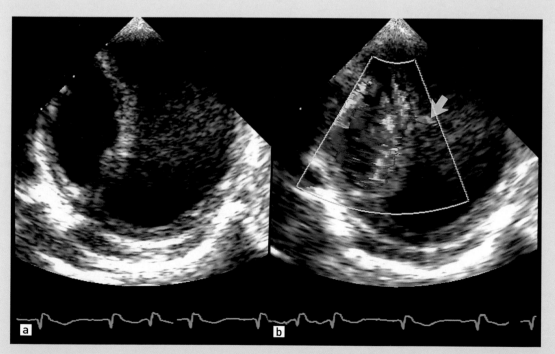

Figure 10.3 Aortic dissection on transesophageal echocardiography. The flap is seen dividing true from false lumen (**a**). Color mapping shows flow within the true lumen with a small jet (**arrow**) escaping through a tear into the false lumen (**b**)

Further reading

Ciagarroa JE, Isselbacher EM, De Sandis RW, *et al.* Diagnostic imaging in the evaluation of suspected aortic dissection. *N Engl J Med* 1993;**328**:35–43

Erbel R, Engberding R, Daniel W, *et al.* Echocardiography in the diagnosis of aortic dissection. *Lancet* 1989;**i**:457–61

Goldstein SA, Lindsay J. Aortic dissection: noninvasive evaluation. *Acc Curr J Rev* 2001;**10**:18–20

Chapter 11

Screening

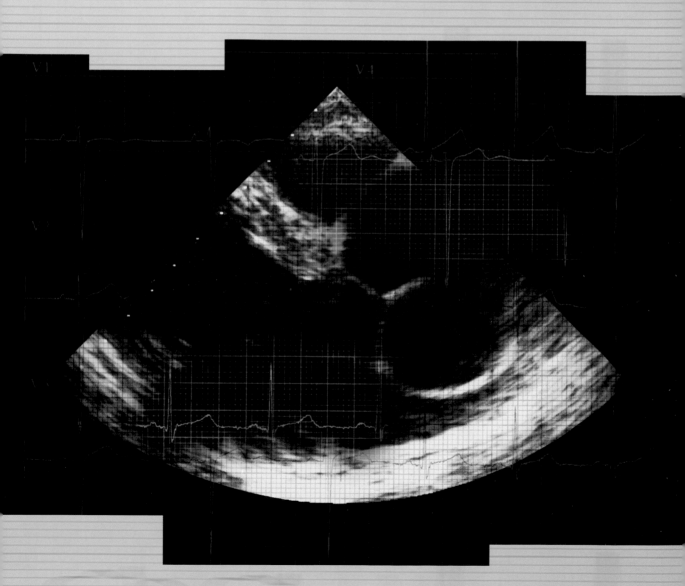

Echocardiography is indicated for screening purposes in a number of situations (Table 11.1).

Table 11.1 Echocardiography for screening
Indicated
• Family history of genetically transmitted cardiovascular disease e.g. Marfan syndrome, hypertrophic cardiomyopathy, dilated cardiomyopathy
• Potential donors for cardiac transplantation
• Baseline and re-evaluation of patients undergoing chemotherapy with cardiotoxic agents
Not indicated
• Systemic disease that may affect the heart (IIb)

Hypertrophic cardiomyopathy is rare (Figures 11.1 and 11.2) with an incidence of only 0.4–2.5 per 100 000 population per year compared with up to 6.0 per 100 000 population for dilated cardiomyopathy. It is familial in one-half of all cases and all first-degree relatives of probands should be offered screening. There is no agreement about the age at which echocardiography should be performed in children. Many cardiologists study at 5 years, then every 5 years until the age of 20 years. The electrocardiogram is usually abnormal in hypertrophic cardiomyopathy (Figure 11.3). Overzealous interpretation of the electrocardiogram should be carefully guarded against. Large voltages in a slim athletic individual may be normal (Figure 11.2) and not necessarily an indication for echocardiography.

In patients with suspected collagen abnormalities, echocardiography may show prolapse of the mitral and other valves, or dilatation of the aortic root (Figure 10.1) or other parts of the aorta.

There is a case for screening asymptomatic patients with a high chance of left ventricular dysfunction who might benefit from angiotensin converting enzyme (ACE) inhibitors. This group includes patients after myocardial infarction or those with a high alcohol consumption. Another possible indication is hypertension since the finding of increased left ventricular mass might lead to a modification of therapy to include drugs known to induce left ventricular regression. However, there is insufficient evidence yet to justify screening these large groups of patients.

Figure 11.1 Apical hypertrophic cardiomyopathy. Apical four-chamber (**left**) and two-chamber (**right**) views. There is hypertrophy only at the apex. A more common pattern involves the septum (Figure 11.2)

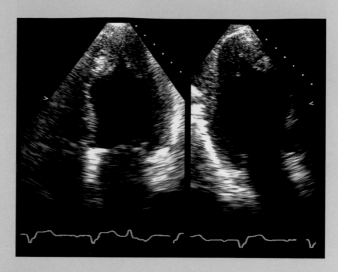

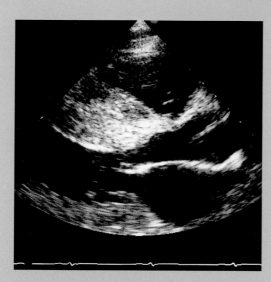

Figure 11.2 Hypertrophic cardiomyopathy. This parasternal long-axis view shows a severely hypertrophied septum

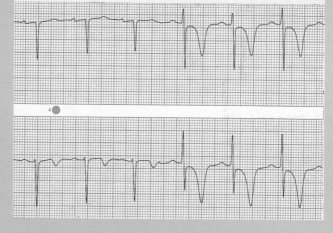

Figure 11.3 The electrocardiogram in hypertrophic cardiomyopathy. There are deeply inverted T waves across the chest leads

Index